DEATH
BY
FOOD
PYRAMID

DENISE MINGER

Library of Congress Control Number: 2013918123
Library of Congress Cataloging-in-Publication Data is on file with the publisher
Minger, Denise 1987-
Death by Food Pyramid/Denise Minger

ISBN: 978-0-9847551-2-7
1. Nutrition 2. Food Industry & Trade 3. Politics 4. Food Habits

Editor: Jessica Taylor Tudzin
Proofreader: Marion Warren
Design and Layout: Caroline De Vita
Cover Design: Caroline De Vita and Janée Meadows

Publisher: Primal Blueprint Publishing.
23805 Stuart Ranch Rd. Suite 145 Malibu, CA 90265
For information on quantity discounts, please call 888-774-6259,
email: info@primalblueprint.com, or visit PrimalBlueprintPublishing.com.

DISCLAIMER

The ideas, concepts, and opinions expressed in this book are intended to be used for educational purposes only. This book is sold with the understanding that the author and publisher are not rendering medical advice of any kind, nor is this book intended to replace medical advice, nor to diagnose, prescribe, or treat any disease, condition, illness, or injury. It is imperative that before beginning any diet program, including any aspect of the diet methodologies mentioned in *Death by Food Pyramid*, you receive full medical clearance from a licensed physician. The author and publisher claim no responsibility to any person or entity for any liability, loss, or damage caused or alleged to be caused directly or indirectly as a result of the use, application, or interpretation of the material in this book. If you object to this disclaimer, you may return the book to publisher for a full refund.

To my parents,
Sue and David Minger,
who give me more love than
I know what to do with.

Table of Contents

Acknowledgments

On any hunt for understanding, no (wo)man is an island. This book wouldn't exist without the collective brainpower, intellectual courage, and ceaseless dedication of others in the field—many of whom are tour de forces in their own right, giants both emerging and established. It's on these shoulders that this book, and the messages within it, can stand.

I'd like to thank a few shining stars who were particularly helpful in bringing *Death by Food Pyramid* into existence—whether by directly contributing to its birth, or by helping me stay sane long enough to deliver it.

To my gifted editor, Jessica Taylor Tudzin—without whom I'd be on my eight-hundredth rewrite of the first sentence. Thank you for your patience, your guidance, your wisdom, and your relentlessness in shattering my pathological perfectionism. Also to Mark Sisson, Brad Kearns, and the rest of the Primal Blueprint Publishing team—for the opportunity to write this book and fulfill a dream. A special thank you to Caroline De Vita for crafting this book's interior layout and to Janée Meadows for the cover design.

To Luise Light, for your courage and your legacy. Marion Nestle, Nick Mottern, Joel D. Goldstrich, Gary Taubes, Lierre Keith, Carol Tucker-Foreman, Susan Welsh, Fran Cronin, Anne Shaw, Sally Fallon, and Sara Light: thank you for generously offering your time for interviews and historical insights. And to Stephen Guyenet, Paul Jaminet, Chris Kresser, and Emily Deans, whose written work has been invaluable for piecing together the nutritional puzzles explored within these pages.

A special note of thanks goes to Dr. Chris Masterjohn for offering extensive feedback as this book evolved, sharing the impossible reams of knowledge in your brain, and being the epitome of a true scientist.

To my friend Lazarus Kauffman for reminding me to breathe.

And to my beautiful family, for intermittently housing me, feeding me, and forcing me to go to bed once in awhile.

Foreword

BACK IN THE SUMMER OF 2010, several of my colleagues and old friends independently sent me links to a comprehensive and scathing critique of *The China Study*, a treatise cherished by the vegetarian and vegan communities for its condemnation of animal foods. The hard-hitting critique was my first encounter with Denise Minger's brilliant work.

Five years earlier I had written my own critique of *The China Study*. This was years before earning my doctorate in Nutritional Sciences from the University of Connecticut and beginning my career as a professional research scientist at the University of Illinois. I was just twenty-three years old at the time, fresh out of college. I had spent two of my undergraduate years as a vegetarian and later as a vegan, strictly excluding meat, fish, dairy, and eggs from my diet, believing such an extreme diet would be more healthful, ecologically sustainable, and ethically sound than one that included animal products.

Contrary to all my expectations, my health actually worsened in a multitude of ways, only to regain its ground once I began eating high-quality, nutrient-dense animal foods. My critique of *The China Study*, which advocated the very diet that proved in my own experience to be so crippling, was the second article I had written about health and nutrition. I have since written hundreds more, published in *Wise Traditions*, the quarterly journal of the Weston A. Price Foundation, and on my web site, Cholesterol-And-Health.Com, as well as other progressive health blogs such as *Mother Nature Obeyed* and *The Daily Lipid*. As of this writing, I have also published seven articles in peer-reviewed scientific journals and have been invited to give thirty public lectures on nutritional topics, focused especially on my unique ideas about how nutrients interact in complex ways to promote health.

In one of the most recent of such events, my troubling experience with veganism—an experience I share in common with Denise—again came to the fore. The producers of America's leading debate series, *Intelligence Squared*, invited me to debate the promises and perils of veganism in front of a live audience, moderated by ABC News Correspondent John Donvan, broadcast live on over 220 National Public Radio (NPR) stations. I joined forces for the debate with Joel

Salatin, a pioneer of pasture-based farming featured prominently in Michael Pollan's bestselling book, *The Omnivore's Dilemma*. Together we challenged Gene Baur, president and co-founder of Farm Sanctuary, and Dr. Neal Barnard, president and founder of the Physicians Committee for Responsible Medicine (PCRM). The advisory board for PCRM features none other than T. Colin Campbell, Professor Emeritus of Nutritional Biochemistry at Cornell University, author of the book that Denise and I had both challenged near the beginning of our writing careers: *The China Study*.

From 2005 to 2010, my critique of *The China Study* was one of a small handful of go-to articles serving as essential reading for anyone seeking a critical analysis of the book. Once Denise released her much more extensive critique in the summer of 2010, however, it became clear that my review had served its purpose and that its time in the spotlight had come and gone. I was so wrapped up in my doctoral studies at the time that days passed between first receiving a flurry of emails urging me to read her new analysis and finally laying eyes on it. But once I began reading it, I could hardly wrest my eyes from the screen or peel my jaw from the floor.

It was clear that for every hour I had put into my own analysis, Denise had put in at least twelve. Yet the long hours that had obviously gone into her analysis were hardly its most impressive features. Few people have the creative brilliance and sheer analytical prowess that Denise has, and yet fewer have the dedication it takes to fashion a work of such monumental proportions. What makes Denise's writing not simply of rare and precious quality but truly unique, however, is her unmatched ability to imbue even her most scientifically rigorous writing with simplicity and lighthearted humor. Whether ingeniously crafted or the unconscious imprint left by her own glowingly positive and charitable disposition, Denise's signature style leaves the reader feeling not only more educated and perhaps even a bit smarter, but having smiled and laughed just enough to make the world seem like a more hopeful and cheerful place in which to carry on.

I first met Denise at the Ancestral Health Symposium in 2011, where she spoke about *The China Study* and I spoke about heart disease. I have since had the privilege to present alongside her at four other conferences, through which I have also gained the honor of her invaluable personal friendship. Demand for Denise's public lectures took off far more rapidly than demand for mine had, which is hardly surprising when one considers the rapidity with which her Internet presence soared.

In the wake of her blockbuster *China Study* analysis, Denise launched a series of blog posts tackling faddish phobias of foods ranging from fruit to fat. She deconstructed dietary dogmatism from such disparate sources as the thoroughly unconventional, pro-vegan documentary *Forks Over Knives* to the very prototype of conventional wisdom itself, the USDA Dietary Guidelines.

She even challenged inaccuracies that had undeservingly reached "fact" status in the dietary communities that most supported her initial rise to Internet fame, such as the myth popular in low-carb, paleo, and ancestral health circles that Ancel Keys completely fabricated the correlation between animal fat and national heart disease rates by cherry-picking his data out of a larger pool of numbers where no such correlation existed.

Through her writings, Denise has earned a reputation for honesty, objectivity, integrity, and a healthy capacity for self-criticism. With this reputation came an audience eager to see these qualities manifest live at the podium with all the intellectual rigor and entertaining humor we have come to expect from this rising star—and an audience just as eager to read her first book.

On every front, *Death by Food Pyramid* delivers. Tours through the histories of the food pyramid, the decline of animal fats, and the rise of hydrogenated vegetable oils provide the reader with a fascinating feast of facts. Self-help guides for reading scientific studies and easy-to-read yet academically rigorous deconstructions of some of the key studies that have shaped our modern views of health and nutrition render the reader feeling a bit smarter, more academically confident, and better intellectually equipped than before.

Readers looking for practical dietary advice will enjoy Denise's tips about how to cook meat properly and balance it with critical synergistic foods, her recommendations about how to reap the benefits of vegetarianism without excluding meat, and her distillation of the key commonalities among the wildly different traditional diets associated with vibrant health and modern dietary approaches associated with clinical success.

Denise situates controversial historical figures like Ancel Keys in context and evaluates dietary approaches as disparate as "plant-based" and paleo with a rarely achieved level of honesty and objectivity. While the titular topic of "death" and the disease it invariably implies may seem dim or even grim, Denise infuses each chapter with a touch of her characteristic humor and concludes the book with an empowering plan of attack to win back the right to a healthy future. As a result, the reader is bound to enjoy a large handful of chuckles and walk away with a renewed sense of hope.

Death by Food Pyramid is as much a criticism of the pyramid paradigm as it is of the pyramid itself. After all, the long-dominant food pyramid is now defunct, but the paradigm underlying it endures. The size and shape of the pyramid and its compartments, as well as the certainty and inflexibility of its proclamations, reflect the negotiations and machinations of competing economic interests, the zealousness of researchers promoting their own pet hypotheses, the inflated confidence among policy makers who fail to appreciate the limits of scientific studies, and the underappreciated roles of context and individuality.

Readers hoping for a tract in defense of some equally overconfident and inflexible alternative to the pyramid will not find what they are looking for. They will find something far better. In *Death by Food Pyramid*, Denise continues using the same critical approach she used in the summer of 2010 in her now-famous deconstruction of *The China Study*, but she uses it as a bulwark against unfounded dietary dogmatism coming from every angle. Within these pages, Denise has crafted an approach that nurtures a profound appreciation of scientific humility in a way that empowers each of us to harness not only what we know, but even what we don't know, to achieve vibrant health in the here and now, and to make that health our gift to the future.

Chris Masterjohn, PhD
October 2013
Urbana, IL

Death by Food Pyramid

Prologue

IT WAS THE CLOSING DECADE of the twentieth century, a time to ring out the old and bring in the new. A time to shift the message from eat more to eat less, to trim the waistline of a country that once considered "skinny" an insult, to unclog arteries and outwit cancer. It was time for a change. It was time, the government knew, to replace the outdated Basic Four food guide that had been circulating since the 1950s. It was time for the solid, enduring image of a pyramid.

By April 1991, the fruit of the USDA's labor was ripe. Three years of drafting and testing had culminated with the Eating Right Pyramid—a symbol designed to convey, at a glance, that Americans should cut down on fat and load up on grains. One million copies were due for distribution by the end of the month. With nothing standing between the pyramid and the eager public except a few last-minute color adjustments, the new guide was almost ready for its grand unveiling. But thanks to political fanfare and a dash of Murphy's Law, those plans were about to change. What happened next turned a federal project into a national soap opera.

Now officially retired, the USDA food pyramid endures as part of the national consciousness, representing more than just a set of government-approved food guidelines, but the culmination of big business, shady politics, and slippery science. Its lingering influence serves as a reminder of the regurgitated, spoon-fed advice most of us grew up hearing but few have dared examine. Until now.

Introduction

MOST OF US DON'T START paying attention to our diet—much less diving deeper than the wading-pool zone of nutritional science—until something forcefully shoves us there. Sometimes it's the realization that our "fat day" pants no longer make it past our hips. Sometimes it's the grim prescription for statins. Sometimes it's a loved one's coronary bypass, an under-skin lump where no lump should be, or that sobering moment when we graduate college and realize that ramen and Mountain Dew aren't actually food groups.

In my case, my first foray into the health world was a cursory one: I just wanted to make it through a day without my sinuses simulating Niagara Falls. But even with wheat, dairy, and soy allergies that furiously rebelled against "normal" cuisine and left me with ceaseless congestion, I never considered that the food pyramid—and the dietary guidelines I'd copied onto flashcards during ninth-grade Health Ed—could be anything less than pristine for everyone else.

After all, this stuff was designed by *experts*. People who'd survived years of rigorous grad school. Scientists. Doctors. Biochemists. Geniuses. Entire troops of grown-up Doogie Howsers. Who was I to question their wisdom?

Though my faith in white coats would eventually crumble, I started in the same place most people do: a state of blissful ignorance. We grow up thinking nutrition is a fine-tuned science—one carefully guarded by the National Institutes of Health, the American Dietetic Association, the US Department of Agriculture, and other big-name authorities with clout and confidence far beyond our own. We spend our lives soaking up their ubiquitous advice, filing it away in the brain cabinet where true things go.

Saturated fat clogs your arteries.
Whole grains are heart-healthy.
Lowfat dairy makes your bones strong.
White meat is better than red.
Vegetable oils are healthier than butter.
High-cholesterol foods cause heart disease.

In most cases, we can't pinpoint where we first heard these things—we just know *they must be right.* The same little voice insisting breakfast is the most important meal of the day also tells us oatmeal is healthier than a three-egg scramble. We instinctively reach for the lowfat yogurt over its full-fat counterpart, knowing that extra layer of cream would go straight to our hips (unless it set up camp in our arteries first). We practically feel our aortas sigh with relief when we pass on the steak and order a salad drenched in balsamic vinaigrette.

Taken together, all these truisms congeal into a glob of so-called *conventional wisdom*—an inventory of beliefs so widespread that we no longer bother questioning them.

That all changed for me in my sophomore year of high school. During a covert attempt to pilfer Radiohead songs from the Internet, I ended up in unfamiliar cyber territory: an alternative health website dedicated to the *80/10/10 Diet*—a lowfat, raw vegan program promoted by chiropractor Doug Graham. The number sequence referred to the diet's macronutrient ratios: 80 percent carbohydrate, 10 percent fat, and 10 percent protein.

For me, this was a "once in a blue moon" experience, the kind of thing we encounter that makes us question our beliefs. The terrible moment Santa stops existing. The death of the tooth fairy. The realization that teachers don't actually live at school. Usually we've spent up these epiphanies well before adolescence, but what I found on that website proved otherwise. In front of me lay the startling claim that *cooked foods,* the very foundation of the human cuisine, were the root of modern disease.

Slack-jawed and intrigued, I plowed through pages of arguments and testimonials that—to my teenage mind—seemed entirely convincing. Our "true" human diet, I read, should resemble the high-carb cuisine our primate cousins ate: a feast of fruit and greens, untouched by fire, spices, salts, seasonings, oils, or anything else inhabiting most standard pantries.

People were reportedly losing weight and curing their diabetes, cancer, obesity, asthma, heart disease, and existential crises all by defying our prevailing beliefs about food and "going raw." Bananas and spinach were the new mac n' cheese. Cooked beans? Their *life force* was gone. Boiled eggs? Heated protein was "denatured"—a word I couldn't actually define at the time, but it sure sounded bad.

We're the only species that cooks our food, the website's author told me, and the only species plagued with chronic illnesses. The evidence seemed compelling. And having already been a vegetarian since the age of seven—spurred by a traumatic experience nearly choking on a piece of steak—I was only a few egg-white omelets away from veganism anyhow. To my opened eyes, the bowl of popcorn I'd been snacking on suddenly looked like a pile of lethal sludge nuggets.

It wasn't long before I abandoned every ounce of food pyramid faith I'd once harbored. After all, I was already allergic to half of its tiers. And despite the USDA's insistence that we eat our six-to-eleven servings of grains each day to stay healthy, none of those raw vegans, with their bright eyes and glowing skin, seemed to be dying of a bread deficiency. I'd fallen under the spell that seduces so many health voyagers: the power of unsubstantiated anecdote and well-posed before-and-after pictures.

I soon entered the lowfat, raw vegan diet with great fanfare. As usually happens when a pathological overachiever embarks on a new project, I followed all the rules—and then added some of my own, just for the sake of gratuitous pain. Breakfast was fruit. Lunch was fruit. Dinner was a pile of leafy greens … with fruit. I perfected the art of downing half-gallon smoothies in one sitting and eating entire heads of lettuce plain. And I was told—by Internet strangers masquerading as anthropologists—that this frugivorous menu was nutritionally adequate and scientifically optimal for *Homo sapiens sapiens*. After all, the brain and body operates on sugar, right? I spent the next twelve months eating enough bananas to feed a Congo jungle's worth of monkeys.

It didn't take long before I realized why raw vegans were so eager to flood the Internet with tales of their miraculous healing. In a matter of weeks, problems I didn't even know I'd had began disappearing. I no longer crawled out of bed in the morning; I *launched,* NASA style. I had the manic energy of an eight year old after a Skittles binge. I started running—even when nothing was chasing me. I stopped catching colds. My skin cleared up. I'm pretty sure some freckles even fell off. Monty Python be damned; I'd found the Holy Grail!

Like most things in life, everything was great—until it wasn't.

One of the first lessons you learn as a raw vegan is how to convince yourself that symptoms of malnourishment are actually good things. During my daily perusal of a message board dedicated to the 80/10/10 Diet, I discovered that my understanding of "health" was grossly distorted. To the uninformed, it might seem alarming that I shivered uncontrollably in 70-degree weather—but as the self-appointed raw-food gurus explained, it really just meant I was detoxing. My rapid loss of muscle mass was necessary for purging old, toxin-contaminated cells. Ditto for the fistfuls of hair I was shedding in the shower. And best of all, my inability to focus on anything in front of me was helpful for staying centered in the present moment, thus expediting my path to enlightenment.

As the months rolled on, I increasingly looked like I'd just crawled out of a low-budget zombie film. Doctor visits ensued. And with those, more knee-jerk excuses when my blood test results came back out of range. "Normal values are averaged from unhealthy Americans who eat Big Macs," I contended, parroting what I'd been told online. "They don't apply to raw vegans."

There was only one thing that could pop my bubble of denial: the whetted tip of a dental probe.

Say "Ahh"

It all changed that ill-fated November when I found myself walking through the doors of my dentist's office. A full year of raw veganism had come to a wrap. I was seventeen: thinner, paler, clumsier, and less capable of forming a coherent sentence than I'd been at any other point in my existence. San Francisco couldn't hold a candle to all the fog in my brain. But I believed, deep down in my fruit-fueled heart, that health was something you simply *knew* you had, even if you couldn't feel it or see it.

The visit began as usual. Stepford Wife-esque receptionists working the front desk. Ten minutes of pretending to read an old issue of

People. Smiling hygienists. The buzz of the X-ray machine. And finally, a firm handshake from my dentist. A blend of gangsta and Midwesterner suffering a midlife crisis, he bore a graying ponytail and, hanging from his neck, a gold cross big enough for a real-life crucifixion.

After a few minutes in the chair, I could tell something wasn't quite right. Instead of the immediate praise I'd come to expect upon sight of my meticulously maintained chompers, there was silence. He offered nothing but a few disconcerting *hmms* and heavy sighs as he skimmed his mirror across my molars.

With his latex-coated fingers still shoved in my mouth, I tried asking what was wrong.

"Wuh's wahn?"

Another sigh. Another *hmm.* Another 80-decible heartbeat in my chest. And then it came.

"I've never seen teeth like this on someone so young," he finally announced, jabbing my bicuspids in resignation. "Rampant decay everywhere."

Even my dentist's devotional bling wasn't enough to soften the blow. By the time he tallied up the sixteenth cavity, I was already imagining a complete mouth transplant.

Little did I suspect at the time, my teeth had likely fallen victim to a deficiency of fat-soluble vitamins—which, despite America's calcium fixation, are some of the most critical players in all things bone. (We'll come back to these issues in depth in the *New Geometry* section.) My mind, however, was too stunned to summon any thoughts of vitamins and minerals right then. I'd been slapped with the latex glove of reality. Mistakes had been made. Decay had been formed. And in one fell swoop, I'd been awakened from my lowfat raw vegan fantasy.

Although the doctor insisted I'd had low levels of iron and vitamin B12, my most deadly deficiency, I would later learn, was in critical thinking.

Universal Lessons

Perhaps I would've fled the arms of dietary disaster sooner if I'd been older, wiser, and less blighted by the bad karma of music piracy. Maybe I would've kept my no-cavity bragging rights instead of spending more money on dental bills than I did on four years of college. I'll never know for sure. But my follies—as expensive and Novocain-numbed as they were—turned out to be blessings in disguise. My experience as a raw vegan sparked what's become a now decade-long quest to reclaim intellectual freedom, demolish bad science, and discover the truth about what we should be eating.

Even if the details differ, the shape of my story is unfortunately common. The diet world is a dangerous place for the uninitiated. When we first step into its murky, scam-infested innards, we barely realize how close we are to bonking our heads on a beam of pseudoscience, or slipping down a slope lined with wheatgrass and dihydrogen monoxide supplements. We assume, in the beginning, that The Truth has already been excavated—sitting behind bullet-proof glass somewhere, crowned by a golden nimbus—and all we have to do is find the right book or website to tell us what it is.

In many cases, we put our trust in celebrity doctors and other purveyors of conventional wisdom, diligently following their dietary lead, hoping they've got it right. In other cases, like mine, we stumble around until some guy in a blazer sells us a compelling story and a box of discounted mangoes.

In either situation, the outcome is the same: we end up a few miles south of real vitality, stranded with our damaged goods and the unshakable feeling we've just been swindled. Unable to navigate the nutrition terrain on our own, we stumble blindly—maybe with a ketchup-stained Rand McNally tucked under one arm—looking for the safest road to health, and the loudest voice to lead us there. If we're not careful (and sometimes even when we are), we'll get taken in by hucksters, woo, hyperbole, or outdated advice too stale to be effectual.

In my case, raw veganism ushered in health problems with impressive speed. But for others—including the millions of Americans who think they're eating well by following USDA recommendations or similar "official" advice—the crash-and-burn process unfurls in slow motion, swerving through years-long valleys of expanding waistlines, insulin resistance, arthritic joints, and other conditions we've somehow accepted as normal parts of aging.

Whether the diet-damage strikes fast or creeps stealthily, we rarely gain the competence or foresight to steer our health in the right direction on our own.

And it's not because we're a nation of bumbling fools, either.

The reality is that most of us grow up strapped in an educational system that favors obedience over independent thinking. We're rewarded for trusting authority, and punished for challenging it. We focus on memorizing the stuff other people came up with—formulas in math, grammar rules in English, theories in physics, cell functions in biology—rather than grasping the logic behind our most important breakthroughs and tracing the footsteps of their discovery. We answer test questions with what we think our teacher wants to hear. We chase grades instead of knowledge. And worst of all, we leave the classroom woefully unequipped with the thinking skills that matter most: how to balance open-mindedness with skepticism, how to identify bias, and how to challenge assumptions—including our own—in a way that's truly objective.

To hijack a famous analogy, most school systems *give* us fish instead of teaching us *how* to fish. That might be fine for a meal or two. But it ultimately grooms us for a lifelong dependency on others to feed us what we're too ham-fisted to catch ourselves. And when it comes to our health, that means we end up hopping from authority to purported authority—sometimes unscrupulously—in search of our next premade meal of advice.

Contrary to popular belief, America's dietary guidelines *aren't* the magnum opuses of high-ranking scientists, cerebral cortexes pulsating in the moonlight as they solve the mysteries of human nutrition. What reaches our ears has been squeezed, tortured, reshaped, paid off, and defiled by a phenomenal number of sources. And as my own story proves, the USDA's wisdom, pyramid and beyond, isn't the only source of misguided health information out there. But it *is* some of the most pervasive, the most coddled by the food industry, the most sheltered from criticism, and—as a consequence—the most hazardous to public health.

The path to knowledge is not paved with hubris. The first step in reaching that destination is acknowledging that there's a vast expanse we've yet to understand. Without that humility, that willingness to follow the truth wherever it leads, the scientific process will never bloom to completion.

Sadly, even when we think we've finally broken free from the pack and are thinking *independently*—questioning, exploring, examining—we often find ourselves sinking back into a new ideology that demands a prompt re-closing of an otherwise open mind. This can be true of those who venture off the beaten path and into fruitarianism, veganism, gluten-free, low-carb, lowfat, or paleo-style eating—the list is endless.

Rarely are any of us detached enough to seek as well as accept whatever new information appears. As is human nature, the diet journey is more of a hop from island to island: forming tribes wherever we go, seeking like-minds, and eventually finding ourselves stuck in giant echo chambers, where the only thing changed are the words that reverberate.

This book is an attempt to unite those disparate islands and learn—from ourselves and from each other—on a more global scale. The only way our understanding of diet and health can advance is if we allow all voices to be part of the dialogue.

My quest through the nutrition world's underbelly has been a sobering (and sometimes dizzying) ride. In the process of trying to fix my own tooth-damaged, food-allergic, deficiency-riddled body, I peered into new schools of dietary thought, running the gamut from cooked vegan to zero-carb—constantly trying to reconcile how such diverse programs could all claim success. I pored over anthropology and biochemistry textbooks, gradually realizing the claims I'd once embraced from the raw vegan community were some sort of bizarre hybrid of science fiction and Timothy Leary fever dream. I experimented with different macronutrient ratios and foods to test my body's reactions.

And finally, in an effort to help other raw vegans dodge the health problems I'd smacked into face-first, I launched RawFoodSOS.com and started blogging. It was an endeavor that, after months of plucking along under the Internet's collective cyber-radar, torpedoed me straight away into the public eye after I published my critique of a book called *The China Study*. Suddenly, I found myself ensnared in debate with its Professor Emeritus author.

If nothing else, each leg of the adventure has affirmed for me—again and again—one simple fact: nobody has all the answers. Science is still evolving. So is our understanding of what it's dredged up. And most importantly, there's no magic-pill diet that will work equally well for all people. It's a reality just as frustrating as it is liberating, and one many health gurus will never admit to you (or to themselves, perhaps). After all, uncertainty isn't very profitable.

Let the Journey Begin

As we voyage through the pages of this book together, we'll explore in greater depth why the "one size fits all" concept is rubbish. But in the meantime, I invite you to approach this book in a different way than you'd read most tomes on diet and health. Think of yourself not as a student in a classroom, but as an active participant in an adventure. My one request is that you revise your beliefs about where knowledge comes from, and who has—or doesn't have—the right to acquire it. We're rapidly exiting an age where information was a precious and exclusive commodity, and entering one where quantity is less an issue than discernment.

In the pages that follow, we'll scour every angle of how our current food recommendations came to be, and scrutinize the forces that continue to shape them.

In Section I, we'll examine the politics—and industry meddling—that pushed the lowfat movement of the 1970s into full throttle, ultimately leading to the creation of the USDA food pyramid.

In Section II, we'll take a look at the materials that built the food pyramid—the studies, the hypotheses, the decades-long accumulation of data, and the interpretive bolts that held them all together. Indeed, many were faulty before they even reached the check-out stand at Pyramid Depot. But before we jump too deep into the science, we'll learn to think like a scientist. We'll learn whom and what to trust when it comes to nutrition advice. We'll learn how to read a research paper. And we'll untangle the complex terminology and scientific gobbledygook we're likely to run across in our quest for knowledge.

In the book's third and final section, we'll take a look at how to transcend both the USDA's pyramid and the dogmatic dietary cages that tend to trap even the sharpest health seekers. By the end, you'll not only understand *how* to move forward with your own diet journey, but also the deep-rooted *whys*.

And now, without further ado, let's turn back the calendar a couple of decades to 1991, when gas cost $1.12 a gallon, Freddy Mercury was approaching a tragic AIDS-induced demise, and the US Department of Agriculture—fueled by tax dollars and optimism—was determined to translate its dietary guidelines into something Americans would finally pay attention to: the USDA food pyramid.

SHADY POLITICS

1
Pyramid Is the New Paradigm

On April 25, 1991, Edward R. Madigan, the USDA's freshly appointed Secretary of Agriculture, made an unexpected announcement: he was halting production of the new Food Guide Pyramid at the last minute because he feared it would be "confusing to children."[1] More testing was needed, he said, to make sure the four-tiered triangle—an idea that had been gestating in the belly of the USDA for several years—wasn't too much for America to handle.

Maybe Madigan deserved a little slack. With less than two months of secretary experience under his belt, he had entered the scene a relative fledgling, oblivious to the extensive research and years of fine-tuning that had already gone into the pyramid's design. In fact, despite it being one of his department's most important ventures, Madigan only learned of the pyramid's existence two weeks prior when he read about it in the newspaper.[2]

But his rationale for withdrawing the new design only sparked suspicion. On April 15, Madigan had emerged from a high-pressure meeting with the National Cattlemen's Association, who'd expressed their disgruntlement with as much subtlety as a whack-a-mole mallet. Because the proposed pyramid banished meat and dairy to the space right below the "use sparingly" tip, the Cattlemen's Association worried it would send a guilty-by-proximity message to the public and tank the sales of their products. The milk industry joined the complaint line soon after, with one lobbyist cutting to the chase: "We're not happy with the way we look."[3]

Even though the daily serving recommendations hadn't changed in over a decade for any of the food groups, the pyramid's layout made clear what earlier guidelines had not: Americans should eat less meat and dairy. To industry eyes, the design seemed to stigmatize animal

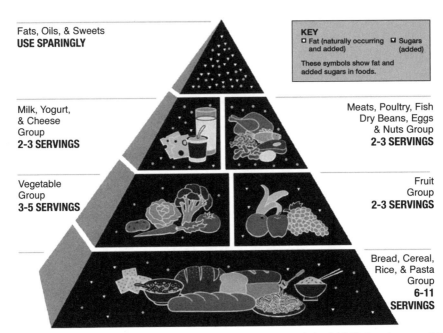

Fats, Oils, & Sweets
USE SPARINGLY

KEY
❑ Fat (naturally occurring ❑ Sugars
and added)   (added)
These symbols show fat and
added sugars in foods.

Milk, Yogurt,
& Cheese
Group
2-3 SERVINGS

Meats, Poultry, Fish
Dry Beans, Eggs
& Nuts Group
2-3 SERVINGS

Vegetable
Group
3-5 SERVINGS

Fruit
Group
2-3 SERVINGS

Bread, Cereal,
Rice, & Pasta
Group
**6-11
SERVINGS**

Fig. 1. The USDA's original 1992 food pyramid.

foods not only by shelving them near the pyramid's blacklisted apex, but also squeezing them into its narrowest band. It was an unfortunate slice of pyramid real estate—the equivalent of crawlspace compared to the full-floor luxury suite allotted to grains.

Upset with the pyramid's implicit hierarchy (and, more important, their location in it), meat and dairy producers badgered Madigan to drop the new design in favor of something less incriminating.

To add insult to injury, the *New York Times* had rocked the barnyard with another strike against animal products just days before the Cattlemen's meeting. On April 10, the Physicians Committee for Responsible Medicine (PCRM)—a non-profit group promoting veganism and animal rights—asked the USDA to swap its omnivorous food guide for one nearly devoid of meat and dairy, claiming that animal protein in any form was making Americans sick and obese.[4] The *Times'* report of the story sparked a flurry of enraged responses, including a letter from the American Medical Association (AMA) calling the PCRM's advice "irresponsible and potentially dangerous."

Still, PCRM's vegan food guide made front-page headlines across the country—leading some nutritionists to fear that the alternative guide would overshadow the government's more "sensible" one.[5,6] The message was obvious. At a time when Fig Newtons were deemed a healthier option than anything containing saturated fat, meat and dairy producers had good reason to panic. But their raucous protests did nothing to endear them to the public. By hounding the USDA into submission, food lobbyists became known as America's school-yard bullies—scheming to steal our lunch money, and consequently our health.

Although Madigan insisted the pyramid's retraction wasn't just due to industry complaints, neither the media nor the public bought his story. Journalists accused him of "flabby leadership," lamenting that the USDA had "saluted, bowed, curtsied, and kissed the hem of the monarchs of the meat and dairy industries."[7] Newspapers ran such unforgiving headlines as "'Pyramid' Topples as USDA Bows to Industry Pressure" and "USDA Casts Doubt on Its Integrity." [8,9]

In her acclaimed book *Food Politics*, Marion Nestle—department chair of Nutrition and Food Studies at New York University, and famed sleuth of the history of American food guidelines—describes how the USDA's own employees secretly spilled the beans. Within days of the food guide's retraction, Malcolm Gladwell, then a reporter with the *Washington Post*, contacted Nestle asking for her opinion on the food guide's sudden retraction. She wrote:

> As I explained to Mr. Gladwell, the food industry had often been involved in dietary guidance, and the USDA "is in the position of being responsible to the agriculture in business. That is their job. Nutrition isn't their job."[10]

As soon as Nestle's comments appeared in print, her office in-box exploded with anonymous internal letters from USDA employees—both hand-delivered and faxed from Washington DC hotels. It was like a page out of a spy novel: unmarked envelopes with no return address, copies of the abandoned pyramid, private department memos, and other juicy bits of pyramid memoranda landed in Nestle's hands, all suggesting that industry pressure (rather than confused children) was the real reason the pyramid faced its abrupt yanking.[11]

By April 1992, a full year after the national food guide drama first unraveled, Madigan was back in the spotlight—this time to announce, somewhat bashfully, that he was approving the same pyramid he'd so overtly rejected. After sopping up $855,000 in tax dollars, hosting twenty-nine focus groups in five cities, testing 415 potential designs, and clogging media outlets with ongoing gossip about the food guide's progress, the USDA confirmed what it had concluded the year prior: the pyramid was the most effective symbol for teaching Americans what they should be eating.[12]

Although Madigan didn't see anything regrettable about leading the USDA through a giant, expensive loop of retraced footsteps, he was alone in his optimism. The chairman of the Senate Agriculture Committee gave Madigan a verbal lashing, declaring that it "doesn't matter whether USDA picks a pyramid, a bowl, or an upside-down ketchup bottle … the USDA's delay cost nearly $1 million and the administration ended up right where they started."[13] Others questioned Madigan's claim that the past year had been one of much hard work for the USDA, since the new food pyramid seemed nearly identical to the one that would have been released originally.[14]

It was true: after so much retesting, the new food guide's main changes were subtle and cosmetic. Spaghetti noodles replaced a macaroni bowl. White chopsticks stood in for green ones. A cheese wedge acquired holes to convey its Swiss heritage. And due to complaints from Kraft Foods, which had dibs on the "eating right" slogan for its own products, the USDA also dropped "Eating Right" from the pyramid's title and christened it the Food Guide Pyramid—a name that would soon become a household phrase.[15]

The image's trivial tweaks—thirty-three in all—failed to reveal what those copious tax dollars really paid for.[16] As the public saw it, the government had spent a year doing what any third grader could have accomplished with a few crayons and some slightly prodigious motor skills.

But the most noteworthy change wasn't even visible on paper: it was the meat and dairy industries' newfound silence. Gone were the "stigmatization" protests that had plagued national headlines in months prior. Although the extra year of research left the new and improved food guide looking more like a spot-the-difference cartoon than a legitimate revision, it had undergone enough consumer testing to prove, to food industry satisfaction, that Americans wouldn't be boycotting their beloved meat and dairy. Burgers would still hit

SWEDE BEGINNINGS

When it comes to things America stole from Sweden, the list doesn't end at IKEA and Ingrid Bergman—the pyramid-shaped food guide also has Swedish origins.

The story is one of desperation. In 1972, the streets of Stockholm were abuzz with chants of *Vi vill ha billigare mat* ("We want cheaper food!") and *Priserna stiger, Palme tiger* ("Prices are rising, Palme is silent!"). Over six thousand demonstrators had gathered in Sergel Square to protest Sweden's soaring food prices, demanding that Olof Palme, the country's Prime Minister, do something to deflate costs.[28]

In response, Anna-Britt Agnsäter—cookbook author and head of a prominent test kitchen in Sweden—designed a guide to help Swedes stay well fed without breaking the bank. In 1974, she published the world's first food pyramid: a three-tiered triangle with cheap commodities like bread, potatoes, pasta, margarine, and milk at the base; supplementary fruits and vegetables in the middle; and pricier meat products at the apex. From the bottom tier alone, citizens could meet the majority of their daily protein needs and half their requirement for calcium and iron—all for less than three Swedish kronor a day (about 70 cents in the US at the time).[29]

Although the Swedish pyramid focused on addressing cost issues rather than disease prevention, it bore an eerie resemblance to the American pyramid that would emerge nearly two decades later. And just as critics would warn of the starch-based USDA pyramid, critics of the Swedish pyramid complained that the emphasis on bread and cereals would promote national obesity.[30]

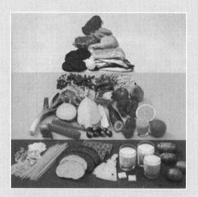

Fig. 2.
Source: Published in the Swedish *Vår Kokbok* (*Our Cookbook*) in 1975.

summertime grills. Milk would still keep morning Cheerios afloat. Tofu would, for at least a few more years, remain an ostracized relic of the hippie. Although lobbyists insisted they would've preferred a different design—and their approval was probably born more of exhaustion than enthusiasm—they ultimately surrendered the fight. "We can certainly live with the pyramid," the National Milk Producers' Federation said in a *New York Times* article, finally nailing shut a year's worth of drama.[17]

To anyone who'd been following the saga, the pyramid's release marked the triumph of public health over shady politics, or so it seemed. The lowfat, grain-based guidelines that threatened meat and dairy producers would surely cure America's ails—and despite initially caving to industry demands, the USDA had taken the high road by sticking with its pyramid in the face of opposition. The new menu, with promises of cleaner arteries and smaller pant sizes, would soon sweep the nation: six to eleven daily servings of grains, three to five servings of vegetables, two to four servings of fruit, two to three servings of meat and beans, two to three servings of dairy, and as few oils and sweets as the country could manage without declaring total asceticism. It seemed the road to health was paved not only with good intentions, but also with pasta.

It didn't take long before newspapers were rife with backlash. An article in the *Shopper Report* noted that consumers generally saw the pyramid as "upside down and a waste of money," with its apex-placement of undesirable foods seeming counterintuitive and confusing.[18] The foodservice publication *Restaurants and Institutions* claimed the pyramid had unwittingly turned some consumers into "obsessive, guilt-ridden phobics who shuttled from one 'good' food to another," and who "impulse-ate or binged on non-nutritious foods" between health kicks.[19]

Reflecting on the one-year anniversary of the pyramid's release, *Washington Post* journalist Candy Sagon didn't pull any punches. "Think about this," she wrote in one outspoken piece. "The Egyptians built pyramids for dead people. A year ago, the US Department of Agriculture chose a pyramid for its food guide. Is there a message here?" Disturbed by what she considered impossibly high servings for cereal products, she pondered "just how powerful the grain grower's lobby was during the pyramid's design phase."[20]

The criticisms weren't limited to newspaper rants, either: the pyramid also found itself lambasted in scientific journals. Some experts argued that pushing all fats into the pyramid's "use sparingly" tip would rob the American diet of essential fatty acids.[21] Others felt the pyramid's unabashedly grainy foundation—with guidelines so vague that a Toaster Strudel seemed on par with a bowl of wild rice—would raise triglycerides, reduce "good" cholesterol, and perhaps be the kiss of death for America's already precarious heart health.[22] In a paper published in the *Journal of the American Medical Association,* a non-profit vegan group correctly (if not unbiasedly) noted that the pyramid's dairy requirement was unfair to the millions of Americans with lactose intolerance, and that alternative sources of calcium should be highlighted.[23]

In 1994, the pyramid's credibility took another clobbering when the *Journal of the American Dietetic Association* ran an article called "How to Put the Food Guide Pyramid into Practice." Written to help dietitians convey the pyramid's principles to their clients, the article would've slipped unobtrusively into the annals of history if not for one eyebrow-raising graphic: the "Hard to Place Foods" pyramid.

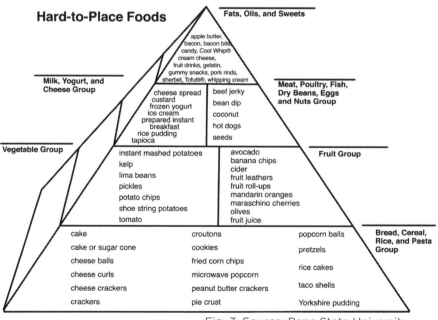

Fig. 3. Source: Penn State University

Originally published as part of Penn State's *Pyramid Packet,* the Hard-to-Place Foods guide was supposed to help the public figure out where a variety of ambiguous items—oddities like popcorn and bean dip, for instance—fell in the Food Guide Pyramid. Unfortunately, any confusion the graphic resolved would be short lived. Cake, sugar cones, cheese curls, cookies, fried corn chips, pie crust, and Yorkshire pudding could all guiltlessly count toward a person's six to eleven daily servings of grains. Potato chips qualified as vegetables. Custard, ice cream, and pudding would fall into the dairy group—though cream cheese, notably, was to be "used sparingly." Overall, the graphic made the Reagan-era attempt to count ketchup as a vegetable seem downright saintly.

Not surprisingly, the article inspired a swarm of riled-up letters to the editor. One dietitian proclaimed that she would regret seeing a professional journal like that of the *American Dietetic Association* "referenced on a potato chip bag highlighting potato chips' newfound membership in the vegetable group."[24] Another concerned dietitian, equally befuddled by the graphic of hard to place foods, questioned the logic behind many of the placements: "Why are corn chips in the bread, cereal, rice, and pasta group if potato chips are classified as a vegetable? … Apple butter is a fruit concentrate, so why is it placed with fats, oils, and sweets rather than with fruits? Does anyone eat enough maraschino cherries to include them as a serving of fruit?"[25]

Despite its food industry influences and scientific shortcomings, the USDA's zealous marketing overpowered the naysayers. The new pyramid made itself known—and trusted—by sheer omnipresence. In the nineties, nary a cereal box could be found that didn't boast that sacred triangle. USDA-inspired board games, posters, cookbooks, lesson plans, textbooks, and choke-free preschool bingo cards ensured the pyramid's message reached even the youngest of Americans. Schools were required to not only preach the pyramid's gospel in nutrition classes, but also offer cafeteria meals with enough soggy pizza and rock-hard brownie squares to meet half the pyramid's requirements for grains.[26] Like a Midas touch gone awry, the USDA *pyramidized* everything it came into contact with—resulting in new food stamp regulations, daycare snacks, hospital meals, and other nutrition programs that dutifully conformed to the pyramid's instructions.

Resistance was futile. The pyramid was unstoppable. As one consumer proclaimed during a Dietary Guidelines focus group, "The food pyramid is part of the way I was trained growing up. It's in the back of my head when I make choices."[27]

Yet the graphic's abrupt rise into the public eye—and the yearlong ballyhoo surrounding it—was neither the end of the government's controversial role in dietary issues nor the beginning. The pyramid, in some sense, was only the tip of a much deeper brew of forces, the visible fruit of an underground alchemy. It'd been chiseled and chewed by a peculiar mix of good intentions, bad science, political meddling, and special interests—spit out only after enough compromise to render its mission useless. And the process had begun long before the pyramid's first stone was even laid.

2
Design
by Committee

COMPARED TO THE BOISTEROUS media coverage of its final stages, the pyramid's conception occurred in relative obscurity. It all started in the late 1970s, when the USDA hired a group of top-level nutritionists to crank out the nation's next food guide. Heading the USDA's nutritionist team was Luise Light, a sprightly New Yorker with an unwavering commitment to public health. In the midst of her post-doc teaching position at New York University, Light had received an offer that would soon launch her into the bloody, pulsing heart of food politics: the nutritionist who spearheaded the Basic Four so many years ago was retiring from her position on the food guide development team—and she wanted Light to take her place.

It was no secret that the Basic Four was overdue for a revamp. First released in 1956 and promoted in virtually every health class in America, the guide depicted four categories of food—meat, dairy, grains, and fruits and vegetables—as a foundation for preventing nutrient deficiencies. With its focus on getting *enough* rather than slaying chronic disease, the Basic Four was simply incapable of broadcasting the message the ailing country needed to hear: it was time to cut back on the fast food, the refined sugar, the addictively munchable processed snacks, and all the other low-nutrient items overtaking the national diet.

Eager to help reverse America's downward health spiral, Light seized the opportunity to take part in the new food guide. After the previous nutritionist departed with the ominous utterance "One food guide is enough in a lifetime," Light grabbed the reigns and moved to Washington, officially becoming the nation's new Director of Dietary Guidance and Nutrition Education Research.[1] Her 2006 book *What to Eat* chronicles the nightmarish experience that ensued.

Newly stationed at the Beltsville Agricultural Research Center, Light and her team of nutritionists set off to develop the foundation for the nation's next food guide. For months, they scoured the scientific literature for diet-disease links, pored over population studies, analyzed dietary standards from the National Academy of Sciences, and rounded up biochemists and medical experts to hash out America's health dilemma from every angle possible.[2] The grueling work paid off: Light emerged with a set of recommendations designed—for the first time in federal history—to mitigate chronic disease.

Unlike previous food guides, Light's version cracked down ruthlessly on empty calories and health-depleting junk food. The new guide's base was a safari through the produce department—five to nine servings of fresh fruits and vegetables each day. "Protein foods" like meat, eggs, nuts, and beans came in at five to seven ounces daily; for dairy, two to three servings were advised.

Instead of promoting what would soon become a nationwide fat-phobia, Light's guide recommended four daily tablespoons of cold-pressed fats like olive oil and flaxseed oil, in addition to other naturally occurring fats in food.

The guide kept sugar well below 10 percent of total calories and strictly limited refined carbohydrates, with white-flour products like crackers, bagels, and bread rolls shoved into the guide's *no-bueno* zone alongside candy and junk food. And the kicker: grains were pruned down to a *maximum* of two to three servings per day, always in whole form.[3] (The lower end of that range was for most women and less-active men, for whom a single sandwich would fill the daily grain quota.)

Satisfied that their recommendations were scientifically sound and economically feasible, Light's team shipped the new food guide off to the Secretary of Agriculture's office for review.

And that's when the trouble began.

The guide Light and her team worked so hard to assemble came back a mangled, lopsided perversion of its former self. The recommended grain servings had nearly quadrupled, exploding to form America's dietary centerpiece: six to eleven servings of grains per day replaced Light's recommended two to three. Gone was the advisory to eat only whole grains, leaving ultra-processed wheat and corn products implicitly back on the menu. Dairy mysteriously gained an extra serving. The cold-pressed fats Light's team embraced were now obsolete. Vegetables and fruits, intended to form the core of the new food guide, were initially slashed down to a mere two-to-three servings a day *total*—and it was only from the urging of the National Cancer Institute that the USDA doubled that number later on.[4] And rather than aggressively lowering sugar consumption as Light's team strived to do, the new guidelines told Americans to choose a diet "moderate in sugar," with no explanation of what that hazy phrase actually meant.[5] (Three slices of cake after a salad is moderate, right?)

With her science-based food guide looking like it had just been rearranged by Picasso, Light was horrified. She predicted—in fervent protests to her supervisor—that these "adjustments" would turn America's health into an inevitable train wreck. Her opinion of the grain-centric recommendations was that "no one needs that much bread and cereal in a day unless they are longshoremen or football players," and that giving Americans a free starch-gorging pass would unleash an unprecedented epidemic of obesity and diabetes.[6]

But despite her concerns, Light was the lone wolf howling at the untouchable moon that is public policy. The only justification she'd been given was that the changes would help curb the cost of the food stamp program: fruits and vegetables were expensive, the head of Light's division explained—and from a nutritional standpoint, the USDA considered them somewhat interchangeable with grains. Emphasizing the latter in the American diet would help food assistance programs stay within budget without causing deficiency.

It was an answer that left Light baffled. Never before had the food stamp program come up as a constraint for her dietary guide, and she'd gotten her hands deep enough in nutritional science to know bread and breakfast cereals were no substitute for fresh produce. As she pondered in her book *What to Eat,* the rationale she'd been given could only lead to one of two conclusions: we either develop two different sets of standards for nutrition, one for poor people and another for those better off. Or that what was affordable in the food stamps program would determine what was best for the rest of us. Neither could be justified on scientific or ethical grounds.

What's more, Light did not believe she'd been given the full story about what had happened. "Intuitively, I knew I was being 'played,'" she wrote decades later.

The rest of her team, powerless to reverse the changes without risking their careers, signed off on the warped food guide—officially laying the foundation for what would later become America's most famous pyramid.

The USDA: A Slave to Two Masters

Although the corruption Light witnessed was disturbing, it was also inevitable. Asking the Department of Agriculture to promote healthy eating was like asking Jack Daniels to promote responsible drinking: the advice could only come packaged with a wink, a nudge, and a complementary shot glass. As the appointed guardian for all things agriculture, the USDA wasn't in a position to discourage food sales; yet its anomalous duty to improve America's eating habits called for that very feat. Should the Department tackle the country's health crisis by whirling caution tape around the corn-syruped, refined-floured foods it was supposed to endorse? Or should it support farmers by boosting consumption of the most lucrative—but often least healthy—agricultural products? A walk through any grocery store proves how that turned out!

To the USDA's credit, its mission wasn't always such a Catch-22. When President Lincoln signed the Department of Agriculture into existence in 1862, agricultural profits weren't at odds with human health, and food education naturally aligned with the USDA's original duty to "disseminate useful information on subjects connected with agriculture."[7] The American menu, after all, was intimately linked to farming output. Greater variety in the diet meant better health for humans. And with nutritional science still in its dark ages, the only "useful information" the USDA could broadcast about food was to eat plenty of it.

A Brief History of the Food Guide Universe

By the time the Department published its first-ever duo of food guides—a pamphlet called *Food For Young Children* released in 1916, quickly followed by *How to Select Food* for the post-toddling crowd—the *eat more* mantra was still a boon for public health. Malnutrition remained a major threat, heart disease had only recently entered the medical vocabulary, and the term "obesity epidemic" was used exclusively in reference to cattle.[8] In order to protect against the most relevant health threats of the time, those early guides advised Americans to eat liberally from every delicious shade of the dietary rainbow, including categories called "sugars and sugary foods" and "fats or fatty foods."[9] Butter, in fact, enjoyed several decades as its own food group—one considered nourishing and indispensible for physical vitality.

During the Great Depression, the USDA continued rooting for Team Human Health by publishing shopping guides for four different cost levels, helping Americans eat well even in the midst of financial strife.[11] And when wartime rationing dented the food supply in the 1940s, the USDA delivered a brand new set of recommendations to thwart malnutrition and keep Americans in fighting shape. Originally called the "National Wartime Nutrition Guide," the wheel-shaped graphic was later reissued as the Basic Seven food guide—a title that quickly proved ironic to anyone who tried following its labyrinth-like instructions. The guide's design included one group consisting of potatoes, fruits that weren't citrus, and any vegetable that wasn't yellow or green. Another group contained raw cabbage, oranges, tomatoes, grapefruit, and leafy salad vegetables. Yet another group consisted exclusively of yellow and green vegetables other than the already-spoken-for cabbage and salad greens. Even the unambiguous butter group was segregated from the group of milk products, from whence butter surely came.

Confused? So was everyone else at the time. But the complex setup wasn't a result of federal sadism so much as a growing enthrallment with micronutrients, aka vitamins and minerals. In 1941, in an effort to boost

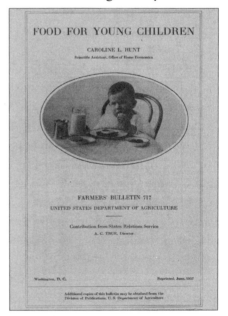

FOOD FOR YOUNG CHILDREN

CAROLINE L. HUNT
Scientific Assistant, Office of Home Economics

FARMERS' BULLETIN 717
UNITED STATES DEPARTMENT OF AGRICULTURE

Contribution from States Relations Service
A. C. TRUE, Director

Washington, D. C.   Reprinted, June, 1917

Additional copies of this bulletin may be obtained from the
Division of Publications, U. S. Department of Agriculture

Fig. 4. Before Pop Tarts, there was food.
Excerpt from *Food For Young Children* (1916)—offering a somewhat mystical description of what we now call vitamin A: "Milk contains a substance or substances now thought to help the body of the child to make good use of other foods. For this reason milk is often called 'growth promoting.'"[10]

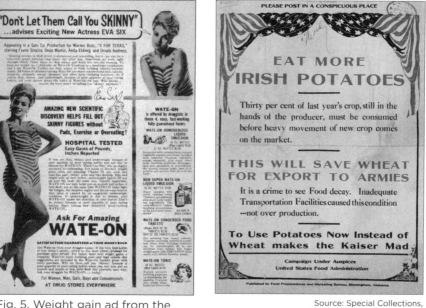

Fig. 5. Weight gain ad from the 1930s, when butter was a food group.

Source: Special Collections, National Agricultural Library
Fig. 6. Food Preparedness and Marketing Bureau, Birmingham, Alabama 1917.

national defense through better diet, the government had released its first wave of Recommended Dietary Allowances (RDAs)—a set of optimal intakes for calories, protein, and eight vitamins and minerals known to be essential at the time. In a departure from decades' worth of guesswork, scientists had finally slapped numbers on how much nutrition Americans needed to stay healthy.

It was one small step for man, but one giant leap for public policy. With specific vitamin and mineral targets to shoot for, the USDA could swap its machine-gun approach to diet for targeted sniper attacks, promoting food combinations that would reliably meet America's nutritional needs. The world of diet would never be the same.

And neither, it seemed, would the nation's food guides. With the new RDA goals in its arsenal, the USDA started grouping foods based on their micronutrient content rather than more visible criteria— hence why cabbage and grapefruit, united only by their spherical shape and vitamin C, were deemed equivalent.

Although the Basic Seven stayed in circulation for over a decade, Americans regarded it with more suspicion than enthusiasm. It seemed the nation favored simple food guides over those resembling choose-your-own-adventure stories. In 1956, after a few nips and tucks, the Basic Seven became the Basic Four: one group for meat, one for dairy, one for fruits and vegetables, and one for grains. Apart from slight changes in 1979 to add an "in moderation" group for junk food and alcohol, the Basic Four remained the nation's visual dietary grail for the next thirty-six years.

But as Bob Dylan sagely noted in years past, *times, they were a-changin'*. As the USDA approached the on-ramp toward Destination Pyramid, the nation was about to face the most significant diet overhaul it'd ever seen. It was the road straight into the 1977 *Dietary Goals for the United States,* the gateway to the nation's lowfat movement and root of the food pyramid we know so well today.

3
Amber
Waves of Shame

ON A SPRING NIGHT IN 1968, thousands of Americans witnessed the televised death of an infant, body no bigger than a toy doll, lying limp as he took his last breath beneath the unflinching gaze of the camera. "This baby is dying of starvation," the narrator's voice boomed. "He *was* an American. Now he is dead."[1]

The gut-wrenching footage was part of a CBS documentary called *Hunger in America*—an exposé on the nation's hidden plague of starvation. From the backwaters of Alabama to the dusty Navajo reservations of the Southwest, the program pulled viewers into a world of struggle and pain, sending shockwaves throughout the country. Under the nation's rippling flag of freedom lay a shadow few knew existed: deep poverty and malnutrition in a land that prided itself on abundance.

Among those most deeply affected was Senator George McGovern, who'd been watching the documentary with his wife and daughters. As he recounted decades later, one scene in particular burrowed deep into his conscience and refused to leave. The filmmakers had zoomed in on a young boy standing against the wall of his cafeteria, eyes downcast and solemn. "When you get to school, what do you have to eat there?" one of the CBS reporters asked him.

"Nothing," the boy replied.

"You don't have anything to eat when you're at school?"

"No, sir."

With the boy's gaze lost to the floor, the interviewers prodded further, asking how he felt about his situation—standing there day after day with an empty stomach, watching the other children buy their lunches and eat while he could not.

"I feel ashamed."

It was a pivotal moment for McGovern. He turned to his family, seated beside him in the comfort of their upper middle-class home. "You know, it's not that little boy who should be ashamed," he said. "It's George McGovern, a United States Senator, a member of the Committee on Agriculture."

The very next day, McGovern marched into the Senate with a mission. He would leverage his political clout for the welfare of the nation, launching a committee dedicated to abolishing America's hidden hunger. He had no trouble gathering the support he needed. The documentary's shocking—and, for the country's pride, disgraceful—exposure of hunger had been enough to galvanize both the public and Congress into action.

A few months later McGovern was named chair of the soon-to-be Senate Select Committee on Nutrition and Human Needs, whose membership would include a number of political big-hitters ranging from the liberal Ted Kennedy of Massachusetts to the conservative Bob Dole of Kansas. It was a rare instance where partisan scuffles fell by the wayside and politicians from both sides of the aisle linked arms for a unified goal.

By 1970, the committee had successfully rekindled the food stamp program, which had lain mostly dormant since the 1940s after piloting during the Great Depression. As the months and years rolled forward, the committee approved a series of specialized "safety nets" to protect low-income individuals and families against hunger and malnutrition, including the launch of the Special Supplemental Nutrition Program for Women, Infants, and Children (WIC), still in place today.

Just as McGovern's anti-hunger mission began to see success, he announced that he would run for president of the United States, a campaign that proved to be an uphill battle nearly from the start. McGovern had already tussled with the Nixon administration over letting him expand the food stamp program, but with the stakes now raised to presidential proportions, animosity became even more cut-throat. And one of McGovern's rivals was Nixon's Secretary of Agriculture Earl "Rusty" Butz—a man whose legacy, to some, was almost as foul as his mouth.

While McGovern was busy tackling national hunger and juggling his campaign efforts, Butz had his hands tied with a pursuit of his own: siphoning every drop of political support away from McGovern and depositing it back into the Nixon administration. Not shy about his vote lust, one of Butz's most prized possessions was a woodcarving of two elephants in the heat of passion, which he gleefully whipped out from behind his desk whenever he had visitors—explaining, somewhat poetically, that it symbolized his quest for Republican farm votes to be fruitful and multiply.[2] And his chief plan for making that happen? Dangle the promise of bigger profits in front of the nation's food growers.

As we shall soon see, opportunity came in spades just when Butz needed it most.

The Great Grain Robbery

The year 1972 gave us more than just *The Godfather* and Watergate: it also heralded in an international food scandal whose impact is still reverberating. The Great Grain Robbery, also known as the Soviet Wheat Deal, remains so unknown today that it might read more like a bad conspiracy theory than a historical event. Sneaky Soviets. Clandestine contracts. A man with the last name "Butz." Yet it's a tale that is as true as it is fantastical—and its effects not only helped seal McGovern's defeat, but also launched a period of agricultural tumult that would ripple through our food guidelines for decades to come.

In the early 1970s, the world's food outlook was a thing of much misery. Global soybean production was down 7 percent. America's corn crop had been ruthlessly clobbered—first with drought, and then by early frost—resulting in what could only be deemed a mass cereal killing. Canada's wheat supply hit a ten-year low. Monsoon-ravaged Asia found itself short on rice. And the USSR, suffering both from unfortunate weather and its own questionable agricultural practices, was in the direst situation of all.[3]

Clearly in a jam but tight-lipped about just how sticky of one, the Soviet Union turned to America with a somber plea and open wallet. Their goal was to purchase a hefty amount of US wheat to make up for their shortage—a move that would become the single biggest grain trade the world had ever seen, kicking off a massive shift in America's relationship with its own food system.

In 1971, when President Nixon first pulled Butz into the USDA's fold, American agriculture was still trembling under decades-old fears. Since the 1930s, corn farmers had been cashing paychecks

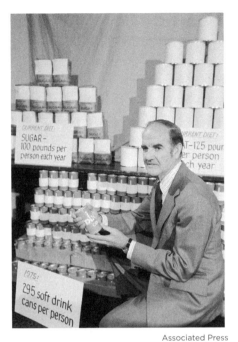

Associated Press

Fig. 7. Senator George McGovern displays cans of soda, sugar, and fat during a 1977 news conference to discuss the *Dietary Goals for the United States.*

in exchange for leaving some of their land fallow in the face of over-production—a strategy to keep supply in line with demand. The pay-not-to-plant system had emerged as part of the New Deal, a series of economic programs intended to combat the effects of the Great Depression. While farmers had previously endured boom-and-bust cycles that shot their income all over the map (too often in the wrong direction), the New Deal aimed to turn those profit roller coasters into something more even-keeled.

Butz, eager to squash out anything with even the faintest aroma of socialism, decided it was time for a change. Viewing America's agricultural system as a caged animal that needed to be freed, he deregulated the market for the first time in decades—tearing down the supply management policies that'd been in place since the Depression, abolishing production limits, and letting the free market reign once again. His selling point—trumpeted loudly to the farmers whose votes he was chasing—was that food producers could rake in more money if they grew as much as possible and sold their surplus overseas, reveling afterward in their products' price hikes.

So when the Soviet Union came knocking on America's door looking to gobble up its grain surplus, Butz saw nothing unpalatable about the situation. In fact, shuttling America's bounty overseas would help push grain prices higher than they'd been in quite some time. Higher prices would impress the nation's farmers. And impressing the nation's farmers would earn Butz the political support he was vying for. His copulating elephants, had they not been pint-sized and inanimate, would have surely rejoiced.

Thinking the maneuver would be a political coup for Nixon and a sting for McGovern's campaign, Butz helped seal the grain deal and waited for his farm-profit-boosting plan to take root. It didn't hurt that McGovern, a native of South Dakota who was born and raised in a small farming community, had already been labeled the candidate of "amnesty, abortion, and acid" due to some of his public opinions; outshining the Democratic hopeful on the farm front would only further tarnish his image in the conservative Midwest.[4]

There was just one problem: along with their above-board agreement with the US government, the Soviets also made secret alliances with some of the nation's top grain producers. So instead of buying just $150 million worth of wheat as expected, they secured nearly $1 billion of the grainy treasure—all at dirt-cheap subsidized prices. With deft timing, the USSR tiptoed away with a full quarter of America's wheat crop before market prices had a chance to shoot up from increased demand.

Although the Great Grain Robbery's aftermath would eventually cause rampant inflation and riot-inducing surges in American food prices, farmers saw their promised profit boost just in time for the 1972 election. And to Butz, that was the only thing that mattered. He developed his own gravitational force for political support, drawing in votes from the Midwest farm belt and earning back pats galore from big agribusiness. Butz's dictum—"Get big or get out!"—ensured a food production future where farming practices could revolutionize and expand like never before.

Michael Pollan best summarizes this shift in his book *Omnivore's Dilemma,* stating that Butz, because he believed big farms were more productive, pushed farmers to consolidate and regard themselves not as farmers but as "agribusinessmen"—or as he put it in another one of his quotable quotes, "adapt or die." Pollan goes on to write that by the 1980s, the big grain buyers like Cargill and Archer Daniels Midland (ADM) took a hand in shaping the farm bills, which predictably came to reflect their interest more closely than those of farmers.[5]

But for now, it's still 1972. And with former fence-sitters firmly won over to Nixon's side, the election became a landslide victory for the Republican party and an utterly annihilating loss for McGovern—with Nixon's percentage of the popular vote coming in second only to Lyndon Johnson's record-setting win in the 1964 election. Barry Goldwater, the candidate Johnson had mercilessly crushed, later mailed

McGovern a political cartoon that placed the two of them side by side, spoofing the dourly father and daughter in the painting "American Gothic," linking them by their devastating defeats. "George—if you must lose, lose big," Goldwater had scribbled on the cartoon.[6]

The levity wasn't enough to soothe McGovern. Scarred and anguished by the loss, he and his wife contemplated moving to England in the months following the election.[7] He opted instead to remain state-bound and threw himself with renewed vigor into tackling American health and hunger. In the end, he still yearned to leave an impact on the nation.

Pritikin and the Lowfat Revolution

It wasn't long before McGovern's concern with diet bled across political borders and into his own life. Following the election, he encountered a man whose radical message would reform McGovern's kitchen, profoundly influence his views on health, and ultimately trickle into the nation's future. Enter Nathan Pritikin: an inventor-turned-diet-guru who'd famously declared, "All I'm trying to do is wipe out heart disease, diabetes, hypertension, and obesity."[8]

After securing patents in fields ranging from photography to aeronautics to engineering, Pritikin turned his gaze to the most intricate machinery of all: the human body. He'd developed a fascination with heart disease after discovering its rates had mysteriously plummeted in wartime Europe. An established problem-solver, Pritikin was determined to figure out why. His own sleuthing—which launched him on a journey through various universities, scientific papers, and doctor's offices—eventually landed him at the door of Dr. Lester Morrison, a California-based cardiologist who'd also been intrigued by the drop in heart disease during World War II. Speculating that the lowfat, low cholesterol, rationed diet forced upon much of Europe might have something to do with it, Morrison spent the early 1950s testing the theory on his patients. For fifty of the most ill men under his care, Morrison prescribed a diet mimicking that of wartime Europe; for another fifty, the control group, he let them eat whatever they chose.

The results were profound. While patients in the control group were dropping like flies, those on the mock-rationed diet saw their cholesterol level plunge and their survival rates double.[9]

In 1956, after catching wind of Morrison and his experiments,

Pritikin stopped by the doctor's clinic for a checkup of his own. The news was discouraging: with a cholesterol level topping 300 and an electrocardiogram showing coronary insufficiency, Pritikin, at the young age of forty-one, was himself a victim of heart disease.

The diagnosis was enough to spur him into action. Unconvinced by the era's standard advice to cardiac patients—to stop exercising, stop climbing stairs, rest often, and take naps in the afternoon—Pritikin plowed deeper into research, eventually stumbling across population studies showing that when blood cholesterol fell below 160, heart disease seemed to vanish. It was a compelling solution in Pritikin's mind. By 1960, after adopting a lowfat, sugar-free, salt-free vegetarian diet and adding a three-mile run to his daily schedule, he managed to slash his cholesterol to a mere 120—and a new stress test showed the coronary insufficiency that first frightened him into action was now gorgeously reversed.

In the following decades, Pritikin conducted a series of projects testing whether his spartan diet-and-exercise regimen could save hearts other than his own. By 1975, with mounting evidence in the affirmative, Pritikin opened his namesake Pritikin Longevity Center in Santa Barbara, California, inviting members of the public to take part in the same program that had saved his own life. Soon rolled in the book deals, the magazine articles, and the television interviews, including a popular segment on *60 Minutes* that brought Pritikin's message to the nation.

Though Pritikin's plan seemed impressive when it came to slaying heart disease, its effects on health weren't universally glowing. As former Pritikin Center director Joe D. Goldstrich noted, when long-time adherents of the Pritikin diet returned to the center for follow-ups, many had developed dry, itchy skin—an outward manifestation of an essential fatty acid deficiency.[10] The complaints were copious enough to convince Pritikin to add a weekly helping of salmon to the diet. And while the program enjoyed success in battling chronic disease and excess weight, its multifaceted approach—reducing not just fat intake but also sugar, refined grains, salt, and most heavily processed foods—was often lost on the public and media, who interpreted the program mainly as a lowfat boot camp.

And so it goes that McGovern, whose own cholesterol level totaled a worrying 350, ventured to California to participate in Pritikin's increasingly famous program. Perhaps it was the "filling but not thrilling" menu that stopped him short of becoming a puritanical devotee.[11] Or maybe it was the senator's demanding schedule and social obligations that didn't easily bend to such a rigid diet. Either way, McGovern spent the next several decades steering his diet in a Pritikin-esque direction, noting in a later interview:

> You can't go to somebody's house and say, "Oh, I can't eat any of this." So I try to cut down on overall consumption. When I'm traveling, I always can order a salad with only vinegar—no blue cheese. For breakfast I can get, almost anywhere, oatmeal with skim milk, a sliced banana, unbuttered wheat toast. A piece of fish for lunch is fine.[12]

A description of his food choices at a banquet in 1988 reflects a similar theme. According to Philadelphia's *Inquirer*, McGovern "ate heartily through lowfat courses consisting of precisely 2.5 ounces of chicken breast, assorted salt-free and butter-free vegetables, a baked potato with a dollop of fat-free yogurt, and a piece of carrot cake sweetened with apple juice concentrate."[13] And while it may seem baffling that a man showered with an abundance of delicious, catered foods would opt for such a modest menu, McGovern had good reason to stay motivated: even rough adherence to the Pritikin diet had slashed his cholesterol to 170, pleasing both him and his physicians.[14] It didn't hurt that his wife Eleanor—who had also spent time at the Longevity Center—was a gifted cook who, per McGovern's own words, "makes the Pritikin diet the best of anyone I know."[15]

After Pritikin committed suicide in 1985—taking his own life rather than endure the final days of the radiation-induced leukemia he'd been battling—McGovern spoke as the principal eulogist at his funeral, celebrating the man's life instead of mourning his death. Describing their relationship as "fast friends, mutual admirers, and fellow crusaders," McGovern's ongoing admiration for the lowfat diet king shone through his words:

> Nathan Pritikin is one of the great men of our time. I say *is* a great man rather than *was*, because he achieved in the way he lived an immortality that will enrich all of us for the rest of our lives. ...

He demonstrated beyond all reasonable doubt that the American diet—rich in fat, sugar, salt, nicotine, and alcohol—was the enemy of health and longevity. ... When a reporter asked me if Nathan were [sic] controversial, I laughed and said 'Of course he was controversial. So was [sic] Louis Pasteur, and Thomas Edison and Madame Curie. You show me an original thinker with a mobilizing vision, and I'll show you a controversial figure.' That is another mark of a great man.[16]

Given what the future had in store for McGovern's own name and image, the statement was strangely prophetic. McGovern, too, would go down in history as an icon of controversy, for much the same reason as Pritikin.

Setting New Goals

The bond McGovern and Pritikin formed had clear repercussions in McGovern's political world, particularly in the mid-1970s.

Although select committees are only supposed to hang around for a short while—just long enough to fulfill their mission and then move on to greener pastures—the Senate Select Committee on Nutrition had become the federal equivalent of the Energizer Bunny: it just kept going and going, continuing to gain power and swelling to an annual budget of $450,000.

But even Duracell can't last forever. The committee—still tied to its initial hunger-solving pursuit—was running out of steam. The welfare programs were as big as they could possibly get, and the committee had little hope of expanding them further or creating new ones. Hunger in America had been whipped largely into submission. And it wasn't just McGovern and his committee members who were sensing they had bumped into a dead end. By 1976, the group in charge of Senate reorganization decided the committee had fulfilled its duties and no longer had a *raison d'être*—so it was time for everyone to pack their briefcases and disband. The Senate Select Committee on Nutrition would soon become a subcommittee with only a fraction of its previous budget, fewer staff members, and woefully little power—a grand demotion if there ever was one.[17]

It probably wasn't a coincidence that in 1977, right before the congressional vote that would seal the deal on its termination, the

McGovern committee whipped out a surprise announcement. The committee's newest quest was to reengineer the American diet—no longer to curb hunger, as their original mission might indicate, but to combat the killer diseases terrorizing the nation. And their weapon of choice was a seventy-two-page report now synonymous with the lowfat movement: *Dietary Goals for the United States.*

As McGovern noted in a 1999 interview with science journalist Gary Taubes, evidence had been trickling in that "there was more to the subject of malnutrition than not having enough to eat."[18] Another problem had clearly beset the country: rather than people dying of starvation, they were dying of excess. It was a trend bolstered by population data and driven home through McGovern's relationship with Pritikin. The *Dietary Goals* would become the first major effort to heal Americans by telling them to eat *less* instead of *more.*

Although resuscitating the nation's health would seem an honorable goal, the maneuver raised a few eyebrows for its haste and timing. Cortez Enloe—at the time serving as editor for *Nutrition Today*—believed the venture had been born mostly of desperation, with McGovern grasping for one final opportunity to make a lasting impression after his still-stinging defeat to Nixon:

> They were fighting for their life. Their tenure was up. But Congress said, no, sorry George, you're going to have to go over and live in the agriculture committee. So to prove that they were really doing something, they got out all their old hearings and pasted up all the things that looked alike, and put this flossy name on it, *Dietary Goals for the United States.*[19]

And that was only the beginning of the storm. What started as a dual-purpose effort to improve America's health and avoid a formal axing soon turned into a dietary battle royal. In a press conference on January 14, 1977, McGovern introduced the *Dietary Goals* with great optimism—unleashing a tidal wave of controversy that, in many ways, has yet to ebb.

Asserting that the nation's dietary changes over the past fifty years were a public health threat on par with cigarettes, McGovern explained that the *Dietary Goals* were meant to do to America's cuisine what the Surgeon General's Report on Smoking did to its lighting-up habits. Too much fat, sugar, and salt, McGovern declared, "can be and *are* linked directly to heart disease, cancer, obesity, and stroke, among other killer diseases."[20] The solution would be a complete overhaul of the American diet: decreasing consumption of meat and other high-fat foods; substituting nonfat milk for whole milk; boycotting high-cholesterol fare like butterfat and eggs; partially substituting polyunsaturated fat for saturated; and limiting salt and sugar intake—all the while eating more fruits, vegetables, and unprocessed starches.

The report was the handiwork of McGovern staffer Nick Mottern—a graduate of Columbia's journalism school, who, while not formally trained in nutrition, had been craving a job where he could help improve the human condition.[21] With most of McGovern's team lacking any sort of background in biology or health, assembling the *Dietary Goals* became a matter of fledgling oarsmen trying to navigate choppy scientific waters. In July of 1976, the committee held two days of public hearings on the diet-disease link, taking testimonies from witnesses who, by and large, were convinced America's food choices were behind its swelling rates of chronic disease.

One such speaker was Mark Hegsted—a Harvard nutritionist and one of the era's staunchest lowfat advocates—who asserted to the committee that Americans should eat less meat, less saturated fat, less cholesterol, and less sugar. Americans should just eat less, period. And when they do eat, they should steer their food choices in the direction of unsaturated fat, fruits, vegetables, and cereals.[22]

Mottern, for his part, consulted heavily with Hegsted while writing the *Dietary Goals,* absorbing many of his ideas and interpretations into the report's final product. As Mottern explained to me in a phone interview, the report's direction had also been inspired by government-collected general mortality statistics he'd seen in wartime Europe—showing that when rationing was in place, with a subsequent slashing of rich and sugary foods, heart disease mortality sank in step. (We'll be looking closer at the nutrition science that came out of the Second World War in chapter seven, *Ancel Keys and the Diet-Heart Hypothesis.*)

Also instrumental was the famous Pritikin, who—along with his lingering influence on McGovern—had helped an Illinois congressman clear up his chest pain and dodge the bypass surgery he'd been hurtling toward. The congressman had been so grateful for his rescued heart health that he pushed the Pritikin program with McGovern's committee while they were conducting research, adding to the lowfat momentum already snowballing from other sources.[23]

The resulting *Dietary Goals,* much like Pritikin's plan, aimed to return Americans to a hypothetical dietary past—one believed to be low in fat, meat, dairy, sugar, salt, and highly processed foods.

Short on time and tall on motivation, the committee's opus was enthusiastic but imperfect. Hegsted, whose ideas had formed the spine of the *Dietary Goals'* lowfat message, hadn't thought the report itself was very strong, and fully expected a backlash from other health authorities. In an interview with Henry Blackburn, Hegsted explained that, given the paucity of time, he contented himself with removing or changing material that he thought was either wrong or unsupportable instead of ensuring that the report's contents were "bullet-proof."[24] Hegsted believed, too, that most of the nutrition community was leery about the McGovern committee dipping its fingers in subjects that more rightfully belonged to scientists—and the report would thus have trouble competing with information dispensed by more "official" organizations.[25]

Praise and Condemnation

Despite the committee's optimism, Hegsted turned out to be right: the *Dietary Goals* sparked uproar almost as soon as it hit the spotlight. In the months following the release of the feather-ruffling report, nutrition journals hosted face-offs between supporters of the *Dietary Goals* and critics who'd rather see the whole report bound, gagged, and shoved off a bridge into the Potomac. The committee itself—cornered by an unexpectedly boisterous mob of critics—held eight follow-up hearings, drawing skeptical scientists and livid industry representatives to the podium. Dissenters ranged from the AMA and director of the National Heart, Lung, and Blood Institute (NHLBI) to the meat, sugar, salt, and egg industries, all with their own brand of disgruntlement.

The report's cheerleaders argued that, far from being radical, the *Dietary Goals* were relatively moderate, presenting an attempt to steer Americans toward a more reasonable dietary pattern.[26] But the opponents were steadfast in their discontentment. One of the most vocal of the anti-*Goals* squad was Alfred Harper—a biochemist at the University of Wisconsin who had more than a few bones to pick with the Senate committee. In his 1978 article "Dietary Goals: A Skeptical View," he blasted the report on every assailable front, concluding that it was a "political and moralistic document" that would "appeal to those who accept pseudoscientific reasoning."[27]

Although it might seem unfathomable today, a number of scientists in the 1970s doubted that diet was even related to chronic disease—and some thought the sweeping changes proposed by the *Dietary Goals* could be downright harmful. Officials at the National Institutes of Health (NIH) insisted there wasn't any real evidence for the diet-disease link, and encouraged the government to take a "mum's the word" approach instead enforcing radical and potentially useless changes to the American menu.[28]

Likewise, Gilbert Leveille—chairman for the Food and Nutrition Board at the National Academy of Sciences—thought the nation's eating habits had only been improving over the years, calling America's diet "one of the best, if not *the* best, in the world today."[29] At an agricultural outlook conference shortly after the report's release, he rebuked the McGovern committee for not considering the negative repercussions the *Dietary Goals* could unleash.[30]

And even if the report's advice wouldn't be actively harmful, *Nutrition Today* editor Cortez Enloe pointed out that getting the nation's hopes up about the *Dietary Goals* could prove detrimental on a different level. As he pondered after the report's release,

> Suppose that, having accepted the McGovern promises and made the sacrifices, it turns out that the incidence of death from cancer does not go down. What then will happen to the public's confidence in the health profession? What will unfulfilled promises do to the science of nutrition?[31]

Since the most pressing gripe about the *Dietary Goals* was its lack of scientific support, the American Society for Clinical Nutrition (ASCN) strapped together an expert committee to examine how valid its lowfat, low-cholesterol, low-sodium recommendations were for the prevention of disease. In a series of papers published in the *American Journal of Clinical Nutrition* in 1979, the expert panel unleashed their collective brainpower on six key issues—the most controversial being the relationship among dietary cholesterol, fat, and heart disease. (The panel also scrutinized the potentially nefarious roles of sugar, excess calories, alcohol, and sodium in a variety of health woes.) As one of the panel's chairmen—Dr. Edward Ahrens, Jr.—noted, the committee had been selected specifically to include "individuals with a full range of convictions" to prevent any single point of view from dominating.[32] Evenhandedness and objectivity were the prime goals.

After combing through virtually every existent piece of evidence, weighing it all for consistency and strength, and clarifying whether any links could be deemed cause and effect, the panel's verdict was in—sort of. Although the experts agreed on a solid link between alcohol and liver disease as well as sugar and tooth decay, their conclusions on the relationship among heart disease, cholesterol, and saturated fat were far less unified. The ASCN series' fat paper, penned by Charles J. Glueck, concluded there was "no evidence … that conclusively demonstrates a causative relationship between dietary fat per se and human atherosclerotic disease"—a deep blow to the notion that putting America on a lowfat diet would be the panacea some were hoping for.[33]

Glueck noted that in prospective population studies, it hadn't been possible to predict who would get a heart attack based on individual fat intake, and the existing controlled trials—science's best bet for confirming cause and effect—had been riddled with too many design flaws, execution errors, and analytical problems to prove fat truly was an enemy of heart health. As Glueck explained, even when such trials managed to lower blood cholesterol through diet modifications, "in no such groups have unequivocal changes in disease rates been demonstrated"—calling into question the strength of the lipid hypothesis on which fat recommendations were hinging.

In the end, the ASCN committee took a reluctantly supportive view of the advice laid out in *Dietary Goals*—mostly from the reasoning that, while there was no evidence the goals would definitely help, they weren't likely to be harmful either.

Although the ASCN report wasn't exactly reassuring that putting the nation on a lowfat, low-cholesterol diet would usher in an era of squeaky clean arteries and slender waistlines, that didn't stop supporters of the *Dietary Goals* from looking on the bright side. Chris Hitt—a member of the McGovern Committee and Harvard student of Hegsted's, who had adopted his former professor's views on diet and chronic disease—took a glass-half-full perspective. He noted that the report confirmed that "the *Goals* were safe, that there were no risks" and that, speaking collectively for the committee, "We felt it was a step forward."[34] Although he may have been right about that, the heal-America gusto with which the *Dietary Goals* began had mysteriously morphed into "at least this probably won't kill everybody"—a far cry from the committee's original confidence.

The Food Industry Weighs In

Questions of science aside, the most vicious opposition came—not surprisingly—from the makers of the *Dietary Goals'* blacklisted foods. In an event that would foreshadow the construction of the USDA's pyramid years later, McGovern and his committee found themselves staring down the food industry's proverbial gun barrel—cornered into making changes to appease not only science, but also the producers of the items they now deemed unhealthy.

McGovern, already politically vulnerable, faced an onslaught of complaints from his home state of South Dakota, where the cattle industry reigned supreme and cutting back on red meat would be economically devastating. (An editorial in one of the state's newspapers had said mockingly, "George, we hope you're enjoying your soy burger."[35]) Egg producers badgered the committee to lighten up on their anti-egg stance.

The sugar industry, too, bullied its way off of McGovern's cutting block through several incisive letters. One brief they submitted after the *Dietary Goals'* release called the report "unfortunate and ill-advised," claiming the committee was feeding an "emotional anti-sucrose tidal wave which has swept the industrialized nations in recent years," and accusing the committee of trying to guilt people into feeling bad about enjoying life:

> Simply stated, people like sweet things, and apparently the McGovern Committee believes that people should be deprived of what they like. There is a puritanical streak in certain Americans that leads them to become "do-gooders." One way of achieving this end is to give people a "guilt complex" so that they will deprive themselves of some simple pleasure in order to relieve the guilt they experience when they indulge themselves.[36]

BITTER SWEET DEALINGS

In 2002, in a parallel maneuver to its *Dietary Goals*-era connivance, the sugar industry waged war on the World Health Organization (WHO) after it released a report recommending that "added sugar" be capped at 10 percent of a person's total calories. "Added sugar," in this context, refers to any sugar not naturally occurring in food; we're talking high fructose corn syrup in soft drinks and table sugar dumped into homemade oatmeal—that sort of thing. The US Sugar Association responded with both fists swinging and both feet kicking, calling the advisory "scientifically flawed" and—in a dazzling act of blackmail—hounding Congress to end the $177 million in funding it was giving WHO each year.[46] Like a schoolyard bully, the sugar industry was ready to steal the mammoth organization's lunch money.

The salt industry also joined the complaint line with its own grievances. A statement submitted by Salt Institute president William E. Dickinson asserted that "there is definitely no need for a dietary goal that calls for the reduction of salt consumption." And just in case that wasn't enough to convince the committee, the institute drew upon a peculiar brand of logic for the defense of salt. While admitting that improved nutrition might extend life spans, the institute warned that "degenerative diseases inevitably accompany old age," and "healthcare expenditures increase if the life span is prolonged." In other words, helping people live longer would only cause another leak in the country's budget—so it'd be wiser to leave the nation's diet well enough alone and let folks die sooner to save money.

For the disgruntled food industry, the olive branch came through subtle but important shifts of phrasing: McGovern agreed to revise the *Dietary Goals* to placate the shrillest complaints without reversing the overall thrust of the report. The straightforward "eat less meat" message would become a thinly veiled *eat more* command, advising readers to "choose meats, poultry and fish which will reduce saturated fat intake."

Gone was the advice to slash egg and whole milk consumption for young children. And to quell the frazzled nerves of the Salt Institute, the updated report would increase salt recommendations from a maximum of 3 grams per day to 5—later pushed to 8, when the McGovern team explained their original cutoff didn't include the sodium already present in foods.

Although McGovern seemed to accept the *Dietary Goals'* industry-pressured changes as a political necessity, feeling the report was still strong enough to be useful for the country's health, not everyone was content with the revisions in store. The report's own wordsmith, Mottern, felt so uneasy about the food industry's meddling that he stepped down from his job, unable to support the changes with a clear conscience.

"I felt it wasn't correct, what they were asking us to do," he said in a 2013 interview with me. "I said, 'I really can't change the report in that way, because I don't think it's in the public interest to do that. People need to know they need to make some pretty basic changes in their understanding of what constitutes a healthy meal.' I departed from the committee at that point—I resigned."[37]

Mottern would go on to produce a booklet of his own called *Guidelines for Food Production*—an indictment of the industrialized food system, aimed at teaching citizens how to implement the *Dietary Goals* and move toward a less processed diet—but it never saw the light of publication.

With the original writer having bid farewell, the committee hired a fresh graduate from the Harvard School of Public Health to rewrite the report, which was released at the end of 1977. In an interview nearly a decade later, McGovern looked back on the saga as the inevitable convergence of politics and nutrition. When asked whether it was truly possible—and wise—to campaign against agricultural mainstays like beef and dairy, McGovern answered in the affirmative, but knew it was a tough road to take:

> The government can recommend, but it's got to be prepared to take considerable political heat and pressure. ... That's part of what the government is all about—to impart valuable information to citizens, regardless of the consequences. ... It's not hopeless for the federal government to take on the food lobby.[38]

Although the *Dietary Goals* made lasting political waves, it ended up lingering in the liminal space between Official Thing and Reject—neither gaining the government's backing as a formal public statement nor being withdrawn. But its impact was about to climb even higher up the federal ladder. Not long after the *Dietary Goals* hit the public circuit, the USDA would gain official control of the nation's dietary direction—leading to a fizzling, contradictory brew of forces for America's nutrition advice, and an even bigger platform from which the lowfat, low-cholesterol message could bellow.

For years, the USDA and the Department of Health, Education, and Welfare (HEW) had been locked in a custody battle over diet-disease research. America's surging rates of heart disease, cancer, and diabetes were sending healthcare costs through the stratosphere, forcing Congress to step in and take action. But the HEW had mostly been sitting on its laurels, resistant to do much of anything. The much-needed shift away from protecting against deficiency to preventing disease had stagnated.

It wasn't until a sweltering August afternoon in 1977, when the Senate and House committees on agriculture were hashing out the latest farm bill, that those research reins would land firmly in the USDA's hands. In a 1979 article published in *Science* magazine, William J. Broad gave his eyewitness account of the fateful moment:

> Amid the shuffle sat Hubert Humphrey, wasted by cancer, with only five months to live. His voice cracked through the conference room. "Look," he said, pounding his fist on the table, "HEW has avoided the area of prevention like the plague, and it's about time that the USDA moves in. It's going to take this aspect of the nutrition program whether it wants to or not." The room fell silent, the issue settled.[39]

It was a pivotal decision—one that would twist the USDA's innards into a mess of conflicted interests that remain to this day. Now that the fate of the *Dietary Goals* was largely on the USDA's turf, they faced the conundrum of needing to promote human health while also appeasing agricultural interests. Although they picked up the activist role with great gusto, the USDA already had a hunch that their rejuvenated mission—to scoot the nation's diet toward disease prevention—would be a recipe for industry conflict. In the late-seventies, the USDA's nutrition coordinator, Audrey Cross, predicted the Department's future with impressive foresight: "We're the ones who run more risk by taking a stand. ... The moment we put out a statement, all the producer associations are going to be down on our neck."[40] It was a reality that, decades later, continues to haunt every move the USDA makes regarding dietary advice.

Nonetheless, the USDA managed to carry the torch of the low-fat message and run with it deep into America's belly. After creating an administration of human nutrition—sitting at the third level below the Secretary of Agriculture—and appointing Hegsted as its head, the USDA assembled a *Dietary Goals*-inspired brochure called *Dietary Guidelines for Americans,* which proudly echoed the advice of McGovern and his team and became "official" in a way the *Dietary Goals* had not. The brochure boiled down its recommendations into seven key points—including "Avoid too much fat, saturated fat, and cholesterol," "Eat foods with adequate starch and fiber," "Avoid too much sugar," and "Avoid too much sodium"—and encouraged Americans to substitute starches for fats, choose lean meats over fatty cuts, limit intake of butter and other added fats, and limit the use of eggs and organ meats.[41]

Released in 1980, the *Dietary Guidelines for Americans* became the first in what's now a tradition of reports jointly released every five years by the USDA and the department of Health and Human Services (HHS). Even under the scrutinizing gaze of industry, the spirit of its lowfat, grain-based message was—and remains— inextinguishable: the report's most recent versions retain the dietary message of the late 1970s with only minor modifications.

In some ways, McGovern experienced a retrospective victory after his soul-crushing presidential defeat in 1972. The *Dietary Goals* he spearheaded became the seed for the federal diet guidelines we still use today—sealing his impact on the nation and immortalizing his name in our history books. Nixon, despite whaling McGovern in the election, resigned from office with his tail between his legs after his role in the Watergate scandal came to light. And even agricultural secretary Butz, the determined stealer of pro-McGovern votes, had tripped into a series of snafus that ultimately ended his career in government just as McGovern's was on the rise. In 1973, Butz earned a reputation for misogyny when he chastised the nation's housewives for having "such a low level of economic intelligence."[42] A year later, he'd landed in hot water with the Vatican when a reporter asked him what he thought about the Pope's opposition of birth control—to which Butz had replied in a fake Italian accent, "You no play-a da game, you no make-a da rules."[43] And in case he hadn't yet offended enough of the nation, Butz enraged lovers of Mother Earth in a speech where he encouraged America to double its timber cutting "in all our forests, including the national forests, regardless of what the environmentalists shout about."[44]

Though he managed to survive several years with his foot in his mouth, Butz finally did blunder his way into his own demise. Sitting on a commercial flight in 1976, the same year McGovern was holding hearings for what would become his legendary *Dietary Goals*, another passenger asked Butz why there weren't more black people flocking to the Republican party. In notoriously uncouth fashion, Butz managed to squeeze racism, obscenity, bathroom humor, and a graphic sexual reference into the span of his one-sentence reply.[45]

It would be the quote that broke the secretary's back, so to speak. Little did Butz know, one of his former colleagues—John Dean, who'd served as a White House Council until Watergate erupted and Nixon fired him—was sitting within earshot on that same flight. Dean just happened to be covering the upcoming presidential campaign for *Rolling Stone,* and was all too eager for some political gossip. It didn't take long before Butz's comment was emblazoned in papers across the nation and, a fatal blow to his reputation, forced him to resign.

In the end, McGovern had—in many ways—left a more esteemed footprint than those who initially trounced him. His legacy remains that of a well-meaning crusader, one who spent his life fighting for the well-being of the country and bumping around the nascent field of chronic disease in search of solutions. Yet the trail he blazed, as well intentioned as it was, ultimately led the nation's health across treacherous grounds. The *Dietary Goals* and ensuing public policy fed America advice riddled with just enough holes to become deadly.

SLIPPERY SCIENCE

4
Evaluating
the Experts

"OF ALL SUBJECTS, that of food is the most apt to be the riding ground of cranks." Sound like a fair description of today's diet world? That quote first appeared in a *Washington Post* article rebuking food fads—in the year 1910.[1] More than a century later, its aptness continues to haunt us. No matter how far science advances, nutrition is still a field booby-trapped with hucksters, charlatans, and diet gurus hoping you'll blow half your paycheck on their life-extending line of goji berries and deer antler velvet. Amidst a sea of voices offering health advice, how do you figure out whom or what to trust?

The fact is, it's impossible to sift through every health study on your own or master every angle of biochemistry in those precious moments we call free time. Sometimes you *do* have to take someone else's word for it. And sometimes you *will* want to defer to an authority with a greater science background than yours. Still, that doesn't mean you should forfeit your critical thinking skills. Consider the source always. That's what this chapter is all about: evaluating the experts with the same scrutiny we'd apply to science itself. Think of it as a mini survival guide to help you find credibility amid the chaos.

Confidence vs. Competence

It's human nature to admire (and flock to) the most surefooted of our seven-billion member tribe of mankind—but when it comes to finding trustworthy health sources, confidence isn't always the best barometer for expertise.

This counterintuitive fact is actually a well-known phenomenon in psychology, first popularized in the late 1990s. Cornell professor David Dunning had been flipping through the 1996 World Almanac when a story caught his eye: a piece, brief but intriguing, about a man who had strolled calmly into two Pittsburgh banks and robbed them in broad daylight, wearing neither a stocking nor a mask.

When the police identified the robber as McArthur Wheeler—an easy feat, given his undisguised face emblazoned on multiple security tapes—and showed up at his home that night to arrest him, the failed criminal was genuinely baffled. "But I wore the juice," Wheeler bemoaned, unable to grasp what had gone wrong.[2]

Wheeler's confidence had come not from his unflappable coolness, but the sincere belief that he was invisible on surveillance cameras. As the news articles tracking his story explained, he'd prepped for the robbery by rubbing his face with lemon juice—a strategy he had endured much squinting and eye burning to test. His proof that the lemon juice rendered him invisible? Why, it came to him on film, through an experiment he conducted with a Polaroid camera.

Wheeler had snapped a photo of himself after a lemon-juice rubdown and found his face utterly absent from the developed image. Failing to consider the film may have been bad (or, more likely, that he simply pointed the camera in the wrong direction), Wheeler accepted the lemon juice as an invisibility maker and stepped confidently into a life of crime.

As Professor Dunning read the news story, the psychologist in him couldn't help but wonder how somebody could not only be so foolish, but also be so utterly unaware of that foolishness. Wheeler sincerely believed he'd cheated the physical laws of the universe. He saw nothing wrong with his interpretation of his lemon juice experiment. Was it possible, then, that the same stupidity that ruined his robbery career also protected him from recognizing his own incompetence?

It was a question Dunning was determined to answer. And with the help of his grad student Justin Kruger, he soon did. The duo pulled together a study to see whether ineptitude protects people from recognizing their own faults.[3] Dunning and Kruger's results, published in a 1999 paper aptly titled "Unskilled and unaware of it: how difficulties in recognizing one's own incompetence lead to inflated self-assessment," revealed that people with the worst performance in areas like logic and grammar tended to think they did better than everyone else—while those with the greatest skill tended to *underestimate* their abilities.

Along with shedding light on some of life's most baffling occurrences, including thousands of tone-deaf American Idol auditions, the Dunning-Kruger effect explains why many of the nutrition field's loudest and most persistent voices are also the most horribly wrong. Folks with low genuine skill in their field suffer from double trouble: not only do they grossly overestimate their own abilities, but they also don't even have the knowledge necessary to realize what they're saying is inaccurate. Although malicious and profit-seeking intent can't be ruled out, it's likely that many of our most zealous diet gurus have a gnarly case of the Dunning-Kruger effect: "unskilled and unaware of it."

This poses a predicament for the truth-seeking layperson. In a world where many scientists seem to equivocate, calling for more research instead of stating something simple and definitive, confident answers can seduce us unwittingly. If the squeaky wheel gets the grease, then the assertive health expert gets the followers. Indeed, conflating self-assurance with trustworthiness isn't hard to do.

So what does this mean for you? Let's make it easy. *Anyone who's certain they're right about everything in nutrition is almost definitely wrong.* Our understanding of diet and health is still too young for anyone to have all the answers. Carefulness and caution is the mark of a good scientist—whether or not they've deemed themselves as such.

Keep in mind that "certainty" isn't the same as "an evidence-backed opinion that seems reasonably correct." The difference is in a person's willingness to consider and integrate new information. Certainty is a locked door; a well-reasoned argument with a dash of humility is an open one.

Of course, this doesn't mean you should ignore everyone professing expertise. Try to gauge when confidence is or isn't warranted. It's one thing to be reasonably certain you know how carbohydrate metabolism works, but it's another thing entirely to assume an untested theory of heart disease is bulletproof. Bottom line: receptivity to change and willingness to admit mistakes are imperative in the health world.

Perhaps Charles Darwin said it best in 1871: "Ignorance more frequently begets confidence than does knowledge."[4]

Who Should You Trust With Your Health?

Apart from being leery of hyper-confidence in an expert, there is a slew of other criteria you can use to gauge whether a health authority is really worth trusting. (For the purpose of this chapter, "health authority" refers to anyone serving as a prominent conduit for health information to the public—including diet-book authors, nutritionists, scientists, bloggers, speakers, writers, researchers, personal trainers, your really loud sister-in-law, and anyone else with a visible platform for presenting their ideas on diet and nutrition.) Though far from exhaustive, these questions should help you determine where a potential authority falls on the wide, nuanced spectrum of "quality" to "quack."

Do they try to help you understand their information, or do they keep you deliberately confused? Some nutrition topics can be headachingly complex—but an authority should at least *attempt* to convey their ideas in a way that makes sense. If your expert seems to intentionally stuff jargon and technical terms into their explanations to make it all seem incomprehensible, it's probably because they know if you actually understood what they were talking about, you'd realize they're full of hot air. The best way to make figurative baloney sound like Kobe beef is to bury it in techno babble. It could be said that the mark of true competence is the ability to teach. How adept can someone really be if they don't know how to explain their subject matter to you?

Do they evoke some sort of massive conspiracy of which they're the target? Quack alert.

Are they trying to revise the scientific method—or exempt themselves from following it? If a health authority thinks it's OK to declare cause and effect from observational data, or claims a small collection of anecdotal evidence is worth as much as a controlled trial, you might want to run, far and fast.

Do they cite references for their claims, or do they expect you to simply take their word for it? Some authorities like to slap down their Credentials Card or cite awards and experience as reasons to believe them—but the "trust me, I'm a scientist" mentality can mask a tendency to play fast and loose with the facts. Instead of demanding your blind faith, high-quality experts provide references to back up what they say.

Likewise, are their references actually solid? Be suspicious if you find a list of citations to Wikipedia articles, tabloids, defunct Geocities websites, message board posts, or other sketchy materials. A decent reference list should include articles and studies published in reputable places. (By the same token, it never hurts to fact-check an expert by looking up their citations for yourself. Once in an unfortunate while, you'll find an article fluffed up with references so irrelevant they might as well have been drawn from a raffle basket.)

Do they get dismissive or hostile in the face of sincere questions, criticisms, or corrections? A true scholar will welcome opportunities to improve their work and produce better information; a crank will loathe the day their hogwash is doubted. If they're worth your time and attention, an authority won't fear threats to their infallibility.

Do they try undermining their critics' credibility instead of addressing their actual arguments? With few exceptions, scientific debates are about *ideas,* not about the people who produce them. You can generally tell a lot about an authority from how they treat their critics.

Do they suffer from guru-itis? A worthy authority won't try to acquire a cult-like following or turn their health program into a religion. Be cautious of anyone who allows (or worse, encourages) folks to follow them blindly and uncritically.

In the case of health authorities promoting a specific diet, do they adhere to a blame-the-victim mentality? It's a bad sign if an authority refuses to acknowledge failures in his or her program and instead accuses struggling adherents of "doing it wrong." Such behavior is a clear indication that the person is more concerned with preserving their image than with actually helping people.

Are they willing to admit when they're wrong, and update their stance in the light of new evidence? Beware of a figure that seems stuck in a time warp and refuses to keep up with current findings, or concede when his or her previous opinion has been proven wrong.

Do they make unusual claims about "textbook" facts (like basic physical processes, human anatomy, and nutrient metabolism) that are unsupported by anything but the expert's own insistence? That's another sign that someone's trying to revise reality for his or her own benefit.

Do they have a financial or emotional investment in advocating a specific cause? An animal rights activist might have reasons for discouraging meat consumption that go well beyond nutritional science. Someone selling tofu might not be in the best position to evaluate the health effects of soy. A cattle rancher might not be the most objective person to evaluate the health effects of vegetarianism. Although it's certainly possible to remain objective even when there's personal investment in an outcome, it takes a lot of maturity and self-awareness to pull that off. Don't dismiss potentially biased information immediately, but make sure your authority isn't hijacking "science" as a way to further a personal agenda.

Do they appeal to emotions instead of to reason? True science-based arguments should motivate you through logic and evidence, not through fear and panic. Health authorities that rely on the latter typically do so because their claims lack substance.

Above all, trust your gut. If you feel like someone might be taking you for a ride but you can't quite pinpoint why, don't wait until you've assembled an airtight case against their claims before you whip out the healthy skepticism. Our gut is often a few steps ahead of our brain.

Credentialophilia

Another easy trap to fall into while screening experts is *credentialophilia*. It's human nature to view those with a PhD after their name as more credible. Letters are reassuring: they tell us someone sat through a battery of difficult courses, endured grumpy professors and caffeine-fueled all-nighters, and walked an aisle in a cap and gown.

Although education is a beautiful thing, it's a bad idea to unscrupulously trust in credentials for a few reasons. For one, there are plenty of highly degreed folks out there with diametrically opposing views on diet—so playing the credential game ultimately gets us no closer to the truth. Once we venture outside the USDA's comfortingly homogenous health pamphlets, it becomes clear that even the most heavily credentialed experts can't agree on how to interpret the body of research they all draw from. If we hand over our brains to anyone who seems formally qualified, we might find ourselves eating a Mediterranean diet on Monday, a vegan diet on Tuesday, a paleo diet on Wednesday, a blood type diet on Thursday, and a bowl of our own frustrated tears on Friday.

Along those same lines, having an impressive list of credentials doesn't ensure that a person is free from bias, or even that that person is up-to-date with current health literature. Some scientists' minds clamp shut around the information they learned in school, even long after it's become outdated; others wed themselves to a favored belief or theory and refuse to let go in the face of new evidence. Formal degrees speak of academic training, not necessarily objective thinking.

The Almighty MD

Whether it's the white coats, the stethoscopes, the impressively illegible handwriting, or the Everest-sized pile of student loans, medical doctors carry an aura of authority and clout. But while an MD might be a far better judge of your fibia X-ray than you are, the issue of diet is a little different. In fact, doctors tend to be some of the *least* educated health professionals on matters of nutrition.

Currently, no nutrition-oriented classes are required to get a Harvard medical degree—and ditto for 70 percent of the other medical schools in the nation.[56] A 2004 survey found that American medical students average less than twenty-four hours of nutrition instruction during their entire school career—with some schools providing only *two hours* of nutrition education total for those enrolled in an MD program.[7]

To make matters worse, many doctors' post-school education doesn't come from nutrition journals or other scientific literature, but from profit-driven industries with products to push. In 2007, a survey of over sixteen thousand physicians found that 94 percent had some form of industry relationship during the previous year—with family practitioners, for instance, meeting an average of sixteen times per month with industry representatives.[8] Even more troubling, industries tend to bait doctors with freebies and financial incentives. In that same survey, 78 percent of physicians said they'd received drug samples from an industry source, and 83 percent received gifts like food, drinks, and even sports tickets in exchange for prescribing a company's products. (Some particularly ambitious drug companies crank it up a notch and offer doctors all-expenses paid trips—usually to sunny, posh locales—to attend industry-sponsored symposiums, where the curriculum is all about the benefits of that company's products.)

Consider this little-known fact: the more gifts and money physicians receive from industry sources, the less likely they are to think meetings with industry representatives have any effect on their professional choices.[9] But far from benign, gifts and meetings tend to turn doctors into industry-bots who resort to prescribing pills instead of diet and lifestyle changes. As a result of ongoing drug education, many doctors jump on the pharmaceutical bandwagon rather than learning how to steer their patients in a better, disease-busting diet direction. In fact, some doctors—as you may have already experienced—seem dubious of the potential for dietary changes beyond the standard lowfat, high-grain diet.

Over the past few decades, industry-to-physician relationships have become just sketchy enough to inspire widespread regulations to keep them in check—including codes of ethics from the AMA, the American College of Physicians (ACP), and other major organizations who want to curb the effects of industry bribery on patient care.[10,11] Unfortunately, even *that* doesn't solve the medical community's lack of education in nutrition. Unless your doc has taken initiative to read up-to-date research on dietary matters and learn from nutritional resources, chances are good that their nutrition education is less than yours.

In Diploma Mills We Trust

Although neither an MD nor an Ivy League science degree guarantees someone's diet advice is sound (and likewise, lack of standard credentials don't automatically mean someone's opinion is worthless), one thing *always* points to trouble: a degree from a diploma mill. Diploma mills are every slacker's dream come true. They supply much sought after—though utterly phony—credentials in exchange for a small fee and simple paperwork. No classrooms involved. No *thinking* involved. If money can't buy you love, at least it can buy you credibility.

Although degree mills have been around for decades, and used in a variety of nefarious ways, they're particularly popular among folks vying for Health Guru status who want the illusion of expertise without enduring real schooling.

One of the more disturbing examples of "credential fraud" is that of Henrietta Goldacre, who received a diploma from the American Association of Nutritional Consultants (AANC) in 2004. Although she might sound plenty qualified to steer you toward a healthier diet, you'd want to think twice before enlisting her services. Not only did Henrietta earn her certification while dead; she was also a cat. Her owner, UK journalist and bad-science buster Ben Goldacre, applied for AANC membership on behalf of his deceased pet while investigating phony credentials—and soon found that the AANC would gladly dole out certificates to applicants of any species or mortality status, as long as they had $60 and a valid mailing address. (If you remain unfazed by Henrietta's background and want to solicit her advice from beyond the grave, Goldacre welcomes deposits of "chewed mice, ready cash, and offers of a primetime TV series" to the Henrietta shrine in his garden.[12])

Other famously credentialed pets include Sassafras Herbert, a nutritionist poodle from New York; and Sonny, a Golden Retriever whose résumé—which boasted his "significant proctology experience sniffing other dogs' bums"—impressed Ashwood University so much that they granted him a medical degree.[13,14]

While most house pets wouldn't be able to do much with a phony diploma even if they wanted to, humans—with our opposable thumbs and greater capacity for calculated evil—are a far bigger threat when fake credentials are involved. In the nutrition world, pressure to gain credibility leads some aspiring gurus to buy their qualifications instead of earning them. Countless diploma mills dole out credentials by the day for this very purpose.

It's worth investigating where a health expert's credentials came from, especially if they already earned some suspicion based on our checklist earlier in this chapter. It'd be easier if fake universities stood out among their legitimate, accredited counterparts—perhaps with names like *Sunnydale College of Vampire Slaying* or *The Redundancy School of Redundancy*—but that's rarely the case. Diploma mills tend to have names that sound like they should be real things, leaving the casual observer none the wiser to their scammy ways. (Encounter a graduate of Belford University, Wilson State University, or McGraw University? Those "schools," despite seeming official, exist only in the land of cyberspace.)

If in doubt, poke around with some searches of the degree-bestowing school's name along with the word "scam" or "fraud" and see what pops up. A health authority who deliberately lists a sham degree is clearly more interested in looking the part than gaining a formal education through a more legitimate avenue. Consider it a high-flying red flag for credibility.

Cyberspace 101

In case you've never tried to research something on the Internet before, it works something like this. First, you open a search engine and type the subject you're interested in, such as "vegetarianism" or "the paleo diet." If you want your subject to be a good thing, you add the phrase "is awesome," "will save the children," or "is supported by a large body of scientific evidence." If you want your subject to be a bad thing, you add the phrase "sucks," or "debunked." Then hit *search*. You now have several thousand websites that will confirm whatever you want to believe.

In other words, the Internet is not a happy land full of Truth Bunnies and Objectivity Kittens prancing through silicon fields. It's one of the few places where quacks can get a platform adjacent to experts, where snake oil can be sold alongside fish oil, and where any opinion can appear legitimate as long as it gets enough re-tweets on Twitter. That makes it a particularly dodgy place for seeking out accurate information. On the bright side, the ease of information sharing has turned the web into a sort of public peer-review system—especially when it comes to health. No expert opinion, medical study, or food claim will escape without at least one blog post or Facebook rant offering a counter argument. But quality control is next to nil. And that means some discernment is in order.

Fortunately, there are a few rules to consider when you've landed on a diet-centered website and want to evaluate its trustworthiness. Let's start with a breakdown of what you might encounter.

Government health sites. These include all branches of the NIH (http://www.nih.gov), USDA (http://www.usda.gov), Centers for Disease Control and Prevention (http://www.cdc.gov), and others. (When in doubt, you can recognize a government site by the ".gov" at the end of its URL.) The good news about government health-related websites is their nutrition advice will be consistent—usually based on the USDA's latest dietary guidelines. The bad news about government health-related websites is their nutrition advice will be consistent— usually based on the USDA's latest dietary guidelines. Don't expect to find recommendations integrating cutting-edge research or anything outside the mainstream. On the bright side, some government sites provide ample links to scientific studies, which you can then explore on your own.

High-profile organizations like the American Heart Association and the Mayo Clinic. You won't find any promotion of fad diets or shaky new hypotheses here—but be aware that these organizations are, due to their conservative and tenacious nature, usually the last to reflect important shifts and discoveries in health research. They can also have some deep ties with industries, so dig around for funding information if you smell a fish.

Blogs. These are websites made of multiple entries or posts—usually by a single author, and usually updated with some frequency. Quality here can range from superb to spammy, though most blogs lean toward the informal end of the spectrum and may be more of a sounding board for an author's thought du jour than a place of academic rigor. As a rule, be wary of blogs littered with Viagra ads, product endorsements, or poorly written content evocative of an ESL-learning robot.

Forums, message boards, Yahoo! Answers, and other sites based on user-submitted content. Use at your own risk. On the totem pole of trustworthy online resources, these occupy the mucky, worm-decayed stump beneath the ground. They're a great place to voice your opinion or unleash some latent aggression by arguing with people you'll never have to look at in the eye, but quality control is nil.

Part of scrutinizing a website includes checking the domain name. Sites ending in .net, .info, and .biz aren't automatically doomed to be unreliable, but due to their low cost, they tend to be favored by less legitimate organizations and people.

Thanks to strict registration rules, it's impossible for anyone outside the government to purchase a .gov domain, and equally impossible for anything other than an accredited, post-secondary school to buy an .edu domain. This means that if you encounter any websites with a .gov or .edu extension, you can rest assured they're what they claim to be—not the work of someone who forked over money to make their website seem extra official.

With one caveat, that is.

Although .edu sites are always affiliated with a school of some sort, beware of pages hosted on university websites that aren't actually produced by the university itself. Students and faculty often get a slice of the school's server space when they're enrolled or employed. Usually, their special web-home is identifiable by a tilde (~) in the URL, typically followed by the person's name or student ID. Like the rat-infested innards of a city, these pages can contain anything from homework assignments to pirated mp3 playlists to zombie-apocalypse survival manifestos. In other words, what you find there might not be up to the caliber you'd expect from an institute of higher learning—mainly because such pages are uploaded by unwitting folks who don't realize their private files will be searchable on Google.

To ensure your reading material is more reliable, stick with the university's official department sites (such as nutrition or biochemistry) and any pages dedicated to specific health and diet courses.

Recognizing Logical Flaws in Nutrition Arguments

Logical fallacies are errors of reasoning that can scuttle into otherwise sound arguments. They're used heavily by politicians, the media, and amateur debaters. Although these flaws in logic can seem convincing on the surface, underneath it all they're like the Wizard behind the curtain—all show and no substance. These fallacies can be used to sell you on an otherwise weak claim or theory, or nail a debate dead in its tracks, or give the illusion of refuting something that's actually legitimate.

The scroll of logical fallacies out there could fill (and *has* filled) entire books, but here's a sampling of the most common ones infecting nutritional discussions and debates. Keep your eyes peeled while reading—or engaging in—dialogues where they might pop up.

Ad hominem. Attacking someone's character (or credentials, or gender, or age, or job, or history, or favorite ice cream flavor, or any other aspect of their life and background) in order to undermine their argument, without actually addressing the claims they're making.

> *Example:* "You're bald and have a paunch, so your research on type 2 diabetes can't be valid."

> *Why it's a fallacy:* Somebody's personal traits do not determine whether an argument is sound or not. If a debater *is* making a faulty claim, it should be easy enough to point out what's wrong with their argument without launching a character assassination.

Anecdotal. Using a personal experience or isolated example instead of a well-reasoned argument.

> *Example:* "My grandpa lived to be ninety-two eating donuts for breakfast every morning, so obviously they're not that bad."

> *Why it's a fallacy:* Anecdotes play on our tendency to trust things that are tangible rather than abstract. But a single experience is no match for objective scientific data on a larger population.

Appeal to authority. Stating that something must be true because an authority—or someone widely accepted as such—said it, without judging the claim on its own merit.

> *Example:* "Lowfat dairy is healthier than full-fat dairy because that's what my nutrition professor says."

> *Why it's a fallacy:* Even the most esteemed authorities can be wrong; their "expert" status is never a reason to let your brain take a vacation.

Burden of proof. Placing the burden of proof—or the obligation to prove a claim—on the shoulders of the wrong party.

Example: "There's no proof there *weren't* any ancient human societies that ate strict vegan diets, so my claim that they existed still stands."

Why it's a fallacy: In any debate, the person making a claim is the one who needs to supply evidence to back it up. It's *not* the responsibility of the other party to disprove a claim.

Cherry-picking. The act of selectively choosing evidence that supports a particular belief, while tossing out anything that seems to contradict it.

Example: Although the researcher has twenty studies at her fingertips strongly linking smoking cigarettes with cancer, she cites only two showing the link isn't statistically significant.

Why it's a fallacy: Cherry-picking requires ignoring or discarding the full sum of evidence—leading to claims and conclusions that aren't factually sound.

Straw man. Misrepresenting an argument or claim to make it easier to defeat.

Example: "The Atkins diet is a bad one to follow because you'll be consuming a lot of saturated fat and cholesterol."

Why it's a fallacy: This is one of the slimiest debate tactics around—since it's basically a deliberate act of dishonesty. Distorting someone's argument to make yours seem victorious kills any chance of a rational dialogue.

Tips for Evaluating Websites

Follow the money. You might be surprised how far the money trail goes even for the most purportedly trustworthy authorities. The Academy of Nutrition and Dietetics (formerly the American Dietetic Association), for instance, has a long list of corporate sponsors including General Mills, Kellogg's, Mars, PepsiCo, and SoyJoy—and its "official partners" include Hershey's, the Coca-Cola Company, and the National Dairy Council.[15] Although the Academy claims "We think it's important for us to be at the same table with food companies because of the positive influence that we can have on them," it's hard to believe the influence doesn't go both ways—especially when the Academy is known for launching ventures that stuff its corporate partners' pocketbooks, like the "Moderation Nation" campaign promoting consumption of Hershey's chocolate.[16]

Sniff out bias. Sometimes, a website's "recommended reading" or most frequently linked-to sites can say a lot about the author's personal perspective. If a website's blog roll lists websites like "My Mediterranean Diet Diary," "Mediterranean Diet 4 U," "Authentic Mediterranean Recipes," and "Mediterranean Fun-Loving Singles," the author's bias should be obvious: they're selling cruise tickets. Just kidding. But such a list *does* imply you're probably on a Mediterranean-diet-themed website and will be reading information angled from that perspective.

Judge on appearance. Unlike the real world, you won't get slapped in the face if you leave a website because it's ugly and trashy. Pay attention to a site's layout, functionality, and ease of use. Web-design prowess doesn't guarantee good content, but if a site is a wasteland of broken links, uses hot-pink text on a white background, and generally looks like it was cobbled together by a fifth grader after a Pixie Stix binge, the site's owner probably doesn't care much about professionalism. Or about their content. Or about you. Someone who has truly high-quality health information will typically strive to make it presentable and easy to read.

Examine who's behind it. Most websites have some sort of "about" section, so start there. Who created the site, and why? Is it a single author or a multi-person organization? What's their background and history? Add a quivering heap of Suspiciousness Points if one person is clearly behind the website but stays intentionally anonymous. If they have something to lose by revealing their identity, what credence does that lend their arguments? Anonymity says, "I could secretly be a dairy industry lobbyist or Dr. Oz or Freddy Kruger, but you'll never know for sure, and I want you to accept what I say as true anyway."

Determine its real purpose. Plenty of folks create health websites. If a website reads like a giant infomercial, it probably is one. Some sites offer a few layers of free information as a means of buttering you up to purchase a book or supplement. Likewise, some sites pose as neutral resources while quietly pushing their own agenda. For example, the Center for Consumer Freedom—a lobby group for the restaurant, alcohol, and tobacco industries—lurks behind a smorgasbord of agenda-driven yet seemingly independent websites. Its list includes ObesityMyths.com, which attempts to excuse obesity as a health threat (and assures us diet isn't really what causes weight gain); Trans-FatFacts.com, now a dead domain, which formerly claimed trans fats aren't really as bad as we think (and that it's dangerous to cut them out of our diet entirely); SweetScam.com, which aims to redeem high fructose corn syrup; and at least eight others targeting the Humane Society, the Center for Science in the Public Interest, and more.[17,18,19,20] To the unsuspecting eye, these sites look professional and well assembled—and it takes conscious digging to uncover their industry ties.

Summing It Up

When you're in an answer-seeking jam and don't have time to earn a biochemistry degree overnight, these tips should help you steer clear of sketchy sources and find the most reliable voices to trust. But in most cases, that should only be your Plan B. Swallowing an expert's opinion without first putting on your own thinking cap will only keep you disempowered, vulnerable to a new wave of confusion if those authorities change their minds or contradict each other. Taking charge of your health means being informed. And that means getting to know the world of science—the terminology, the inner workings, the methods, the madness. In the next chapter, we'll fill up your critical-thinking toolbox with everything you need to do just that.

5
The Hitchhiker's Guide to Nutritional Research

EVEN IF YOU'VE NEVER HEARD OF Science-ese before, you've surely seen it. It's the impenetrable language of studies, oozing with jargon and acronyms—the kind of writing known to glaze eyes and induce narcolepsy. Science-ese is what greets us when we happen upon a peer-reviewed journal article on the Internet. It lurks in our college textbooks. It compels us to sign up for art class instead of biochemistry. And it almost fools us into thinking it's English, until we take a closer look and realize that, despite its deceptive use of the Roman alphabet, "aceruloplasminemia" can't possibly be a real word.

Science-ese ultimately prevents most of us from venturing beyond the reader-friendly blurbs we see in newspapers and popular diet books. It holds us hostage to ignorance, ensuring any health news we receive must first pass through layers of middlemen.

Fortunately, it doesn't have to be that way. Like any language, the statistical gobbledygook that is Science-ese is fabulously learnable—even if you don't have a PhD or years of training in the field. And that's what this chapter is all about. What follows is a pocket-guide for translating the intimidating terms and concepts that tend to spook us with their foreignness. By the time you reach the end of this chapter, you will have learned the secret: Science-ese really is more bark than bite.

THE SCIENCE-ESE TRANSLATOR

Blinding. The act of keeping various players in a study unaware of who's receiving what treatment. A study can have different levels of blinding: single-blind, double-blind, and even triple-blind. And it can include the subjects, the investigators, the physicians, or the assessors collecting outcome data. Blinding is vital in reducing bias and preventing the *placebo effect* (see page 72).

Citation. A reference to another published scientific work.

Cohort. A group of people with common characteristics or experiences, often used in observational research.

Control. An element that's held constant throughout an experiment.

Confounder. A hidden variable that can obscure an association (or create the illusion of one) between the items under study.

Correlation. A relationship between two variables generally represented by the *r value* (*r*=). Remember this value when we dissect the studies featured in the next few chapters. Essentially, *positive correlations* range from 0 to 1, and *negative correlations* range from -1 to 0; a correlation of 0 is perfectly neutral, meaning the two things under study don't appear related in any way. The closer to 1 or -1 the correlation is—say, 0.93 or -0.84—the stronger the relationship between the variables, either positive or negative respectively. Let's use Garfield the cat as an example:

The more food Garfield scarfs down, the more Garfield weighs; the less food Garfield scarfs down, the less Garfield weighs. This is a positive correlation because the two variables—Garfield's food intake and his weight—increase together and decrease together. The value for this might be expressed as *r*= 1.

If we found that the more Garfield exercises, the less Garfield weighs, and the less Garfield exercises, the more Garfield weighs, we'd show a *negative correlation* because one variable increases while the other decreases, and vice versa. This might be expressed as *r*= -1. (See sidebar on page 70.)

THE ETYMOLOGY OF EPIDEMIOLOGY

Decoding Science-ese is sometimes just a matter of breaking down the Latin or Greek root words. For instance, epidemiology. *Epi* means "on," or "upon," like how your skin (*epi*dermis) is upon you. And "dem"—as in democracy, demography, or other words that relate to "people." *Epidemiology*, therefore, is the study of "what is upon the people," or, in modern terms, what's making them sick.

Epidemiology. The study of how diseases spread and can be controlled. Traditionally, it looked at diseases such as cholera, small pox, malaria, and so forth, drawing links to factors like sanitation, sewage, and drinking water. In recent decades, epidemioloy has looked at non-infectious diseases like heart disease, and draws links to lifestyle factors such as diet, smoking, and lack of exercise.

This type of research generally derives conclusions from observational, non-experimental studies that drum up data and create statistical hunting grounds for researchers. And like any form of observation, it doesn't have the final say in cause and effect.

Experimental group. A group of participants (human or otherwise) exposed to some sort of changed variable—like a new diet, medication, or exercise program. When compared with a control group, the results of the experimental group make it possible to see what effect the changed variable elicited.

Experiments. These involve rolling up your sleeves and changing something about the situation you're studying—in contrast to simply sitting back and observing a situation unfold naturally. Think mad scientist with a shock of unkempt hair, clutching a beaker as he prepares to find out what happens when you mix nitric acid and hydrazine. Not all experiments involve things exploding, of course: they could also mean administering a cholesterol-lowering drug, or giving study participants a new diet to follow, or putting folks on an exercise program to study weight loss. The possibilities are endless. But no matter what, an experiment involves making some sort of *change* in order to study the outcome.

Hypothesis. An "educated guess" explaining whatever phenomena you're studying—typically based on past experience, observations, logic, and background knowledge.

Number needed to treat (NNT). How many people need to be treated in order to see the effect of the treatment on one person.

Peer review. The act of scholars weighing in on the work of other professionals in their field—a human-powered quality-control tactic to weed out errors and ensure findings have merit. Considered the gold standard of scientific publications, peer-reviewed studies can seem infallible to the media and general public alike, and often dodge the scrutiny and skepticism other publications receive.

Unfortunately, the reality is hardly rosy. As *Lancet* editor Richard Horton—whose career pinned him nose-to-nose with the peer-review process—once explained, "We know that the system of peer review is biased, unjust, unaccountable, incomplete, easily fixed, often insulting, usually ignorant, occasionally foolish, and frequently wrong."[1] Drummond Rennie, the deputy editor of the *Journal of the American Medical Association,* echoed similar sentiments:

A NOTE ON CORRELATION

If statisticians were warriors, they'd be chanting the battle cry "Correlation doesn't imply causation!" It's one of the most important concepts to grasp when looking at data, and it's also the one most frequently bungled.

In a nutshell, *correlation doesn't imply causation* states that just because two things have some sort of relationship, it doesn't mean one is causing the other (or preventing it, for that matter). Often, two variables that seem to be trotting along hand-in-hand are actually united by a third, hidden influence. Eating popsicles might be correlated with getting sunburned—not because the icy treats make your skin extra sensitive, but because you're more likely to reach for such a thing on days when the sun is blazing. Drinking morning coffee might be correlated with feeling exhausted at the end of the day, but maybe both are related to your alarm going off before sunrise. Sleeping with shoes on might be correlated with waking up with a hangover, but pulling off your sneakers before bed won't stop that headache if the real culprit is tequila. Get the picture?

Even rigorous studies have churned up wacky correlations that clearly don't have a cause-and-effect relationship. And a lot of times, as with the examples above, all we need is our innate common sense to figure out what's *really* linking a set of circumstances together.

But when it comes to nutrition and health, it's not so simple. Different components of diet, lifestyle, and health are highly interwoven, and it's often hard to decipher whether they're interacting in causal or accidental ways. For example, someone who

There seems to be no study too fragmented, no hypothesis too trivial, no literature too biased or too egotistical, no design too warped, no methodology too bungled, no presentation of results too inaccurate, too obscure, and too contradictory, no analysis too self-serving, no argument too circular, no conclusions too trifling or too unjustified, and no grammar and syntax too offensive for a paper to end up in print.[2]

While the peer-review process certainly improves the quality of studies entering scientific journals, it doesn't guarantee perfection. We shouldn't assume that just because a study endured peer review, all the thinking has been done for us.

is health-conscious by conventional standards might load their plates with whole grains, fruit, salads, yogurt, fish, and drink fizzy kombucha drinks—while also biking to work and attending yoga on weekends. That person may very well be healthier than the average bear, and if we took any one component of that person's diet, we'd probably find each one correlates with better health outcomes. But whether that's owed to the kombucha, the exercise, the fresh air, the fruit, or any other variable remains a question mark.

Broadly speaking, the only way to really prove cause and effect is through randomized controlled trials. (See Controlled Trials on page 78.) That's the surest way to mute all the white noise and track a single variable to see what it's up to. The problem, of course, is that it's not always possible—or ethical—to conduct these sorts of trials when human disease is involved, and that means some questions in health might never have a truly conclusive answer.

Also, bear in mind that while correlation might not *prove* causation, it can sometimes be a pretty good indicator that something is worth a deeper look. The tobacco industry, for instance, championed the *correlation isn't causation* message when cancer started showing up alongside tobacco use in observational studies. So how can you tell when correlation probably *is* causation? When the link in observational data is *strong* (think: high risk ratios), *consistent* (it pops up in multiple populations and generally points in the same direction), has *biological plausibility* (we have at least a rough idea of what could be going on in the body to make the health outcome happen), and is *unlikely to be confounded* by other variables.

Placebo. A treatment or medicine intended to have zero effect on the condition under study.

Placebo effect. A "mind over matter" phenomenon where a neutral treatment produces some sort of beneficial effect. Since that benefit shouldn't be attributed to anything special about the placebo itself (at least in an ideal world), it must therefore be due to the patient's own expectation.

Risk. Study results are often reported in terms of *risk*—the chance of something taking place, like a disease or other health outcome. But there are two ways risk can be conveyed, and knowing the difference is a crucial part of study interpretation.

> ***Absolute risk.*** This term shows the overall likelihood of an event happening. Here's an example: "Smokers have a one in six lifetime risk of developing lung cancer." The higher the absolute risk becomes—say, one in three—the more likely that the event will happen, but since we're only dealing with probabilities, there's no guarantee it actually will.

> ***Relative risk.*** Most study results are reported as a *relative risk,* which tells us how much more or less likely a disease is in one group compared to another. Unfortunately, relative risk has a tendency to make findings seem wildly more dramatic than they actually are—and is often used to dress up absolute risk to exaggerate its importance. Here's an example from a real study: *Eating red meat three times a week doubles your risk of colon cancer.* That's enough to make anyone trade a juicy steak in for a salmon patty (or a slab of well-seasoned tofu). But even though a "doubled risk" sounds scary, it's actually quite meaningless until we know what the *absolute* risk is, too. In this instance, the doubled risk only meant that four out of one thousand people—rather than two out of one thousand people—got colon cancer.

Sample size. The number of people (or non-human participants) in a group being studied. For the sake of drawing sturdy conclusions from the data and establishing statistical significance, researchers typically want as large a sample size as possible.

Significance. When we hear the word "significant" in daily life, it usually means something big or important. "His blood loss was *significant.*" "She had *significant* doubts about the crepe recipe." "He spent a *significant* amount of time playing Kitten Cannonball before his boss checked his browser history and moved him to the sales floor." That's all well and good—but when it comes to scientific reporting, the term "significant" has a much different meaning.

Statistically significant. In statistics, *significant* only means that the results at hand are unlikely due to chance. It doesn't imply those results are particularly momentous, and it doesn't ensure the numbers aren't confounded by something the scientists didn't measure (or that they measured inaccurately). All it means is that mathematically, the results are probably not an accident.

For instance, a study might say that "eating pie significantly increases your risk of a stroke," but a closer look at the findings could reveal that pie consumption was associated with an increase of stroke from 3 percent to 3.2 percent. In this case, that increase is mathematically significant, but perhaps not *clinically* significant—meaning the finding at hand probably isn't anything to change your life over.

In studies (and math at large), statistical significance is represented by something called a *p value* ($p=$). You'll see references to the p value in tables and charts, and scattered throughout the Results and Discussion section of most scientific studies. The p value is a measure of how likely it is that a relationship you found within your data was just luck of the draw, rather than representing something meaningful—for instance, flipping a coin three times in a row and getting tails each time. Most scientists draw the line at a p value of 0.05, with lower values indicating less likelihood that your results were due to chance.

Clinically significant. This is the term we're looking for when we want to say something matters in the real world. If a study finds that avoiding Skittles will slash your risk of choking by 20 percent (perhaps a *statistically significant* finding) but that it'd take forty thousand folks vowing Skittle-abstinence to actually make that happen, we have a finding that's not clinically meaningful; any anti-Skittle treatment won't make a big impact on the world. On the flip side, if a study finds that a diet intervention would prevent a heart attack in three out of five at-risk patients with cardiovascular disease, that's some top-notch *clinical significance* right there.

Variable. Any factor that can be controlled or changed in an experiment—like diet, medication, daily exercise, and so forth. An *independent variable* is the one condition you change in an experiment, while a *dependent variable* is the thing you measure or observe.

Types of Studies

By now, you've probably stumbled on a universal truth: not all studies are created equal. Luckily, there are ways to figure out in a snap how much stock we should put in the latest dietary findings by knowing how a particular study was designed and how its data was collected. Let's take a look at some of the more common types of research, starting from the least relevant down to the most relevant for human nutrition.

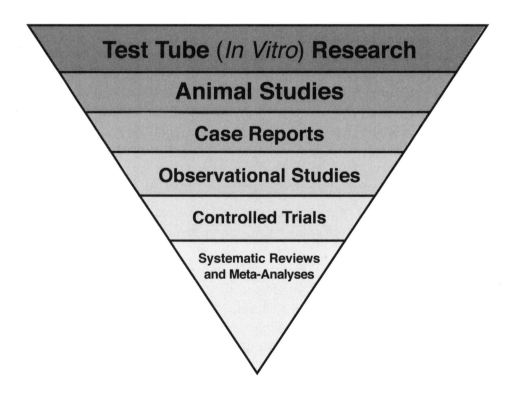

Test Tube (In Vitro) Research

The word *in vitro* means "within the glass"—which pretty much sums up this form of research. Rather than taking place in a living organism, *in vitro* research happens in a test tube or petri dish, where scientists can isolate specific cells, viruses, or bacteria and study them outside of the biological system they came from. While it's a great way to gain mechanistic insights (not to mention bypass the ethical hurdles of human research), *in vitro* studies rarely apply to real life: glass tubes are just no match for the complexity of a living organism.

Animal Studies

Love of cheese notwithstanding, humans and mice have some significant differences. Same goes for the other critters often used in research intended to shed light on human health and disease. While animal studies can be useful for venturing where no human study dare go— whether due to impracticality or riskiness or ethical qualms—they can also be grossly misleading.

The biggest problem comes when trying to extrapolate the effects of lab diets to anything relevant for humans. Case in point, the following culinary masterpiece is actually the standard American diet formula for rodents, from Purina Test Diets—frequently used as the "high-fat diet" in those mouse studies we read about in the news.[3]

- Cornstarch
- Casein
- Maltodextrin
- Sucrose
- Vegetable shortening
- Milk fat
- Lard
- AIN93G Mineral Mix/Fiber
- Powdered cellulose
- Inulin
- Soybean oil
- AIN93 Vitamin Mix/Fiber
- Corn oil
- L-Cystine
- Choline bitartrate
- Cholesterol
- FD&C Red 40 Lake

Go ahead and look at that list of ingredients again. When a rodent study comes out saying a high-fat diet causes diabetes, heart disease, cancer, osteoporosis, or Alzheimer's, *this* is usually the diet they're talking about. Perhaps you can see the problem with generalizing the findings of such studies to actual humans who eat people food.

Even worse, we can't just blame the media's discombobulator machine for the rampant abuse of mouse studies. Many researchers themselves are quick to draw conclusions about the human diet based on hyper-processed lumps of Crisco, sucrose, and cornstarch fed to creatures the size of our palm.

In 2008, two researchers from UC Davis conducted a literature review of studies containing the keywords "mouse high fat" published in high-impact journals during the year before.[4] Of the thirty-five papers surveyed, only five compared diets with identical nutrients that differed only in fat and carbohydrate content; the other thirty either inappropriately compared chow with purified high-fat diets, or didn't provide enough information to tell what was going on diet-wise.

As the UC Davis researchers noted, the difference between "high fat" test diets and regular mouse chow is more than a matter of mac-ronutrients.

"Regular chow," which scientists often use for the control group in high-fat-diet mouse studies, is made from actual foods you might find in a human diet: ground wheat, oats, corn, alfalfa meal, fish, and fats from vegetable sources, among other agricultural byproducts.

By contrast, "purified diets" merely *mimic* a high-fat human diet, and are made up of an assortment of refined ingredients: typically the milk protein casein, cornstarch, a sugar-like sucrose or maltodextrin, a fat-like soybean oil or lard, and a vitamin and mineral complex to round it all out.

The UC Davis researchers noted that the chow diet versus the purified diet can differ in phytoestrogen content—potentially influencing food and water intake, learning, memory, insulin levels, leptin levels, thyroid levels, anxiety, the creation or breakdown of fat, and other characteristics sometimes serving as the study's very focus.

So when a news story says something like "High-fat diet in mice causes [terrible illness]," it really means researchers fed mice a diet of soybean oil, hydrogenated coconut oil, sugar, and maltodextrin to make them obese, and then studied the effects of that obesity. Fact is, animal studies, on rodents in particular, are *not* about elucidating the links between what humans eat and the sicknesses that befall us, even if reported that way. A rat study will never have bearing on your life, because unlike lab animals, you are not eating a purified diet of sucrose, corn oil, casein, and synthetic vitamins from birth until death.

Case Reports

These describe or analyze a person, a group, or a unique situation. You find them once in a while in news headlines. The title might read something like "Child born B-12 deficient from fruitarian mother," or "Man survives fourteen years with nail lodged in his skull." Although some case studies can be pretty interesting, they aren't capable of unraveling any great, generalized truths about the universe and its innermost workings. You can read them for entertainment value, but this type of study probably won't have any significant application to your life (unless, of course, you *are* the case study). Simply put, a study of one just doesn't provide a big enough sample size to draw conclusions about the rest of the population.

Observational Studies

This form of research exists to describe patterns and trends—observing a situation unobtrusively, without asking people to change anything about their diet or lifestyle or medications. Although observational studies can be useful for finding leads for controlled studies, basing your nutritional worldview on an observational study would be like a detective trying to solve a murder with nothing but a photo of the crime scene. Without dusting for fingerprints, testing DNA and hair samples, interviewing suspects, and otherwise delving deeper into the situation, it'd be easy to reach the wrong conclusion. ("Ah, see how he collapsed right next to that lamp? It was the incandescent light that did him in!") This type of research is the breeding ground, too, for mistaking correlation for causation (see page 70). While observational studies are a good place to start, they are *never* a good place to stop.

It's pretty easy to spot an observational study in a news report. If an article says something like "Researchers followed 400 vegetarians for 10 years..." or "Scientists find greater number of 'above average' residents in Lake Woebegone than any other American city," those are clues the study at hand is observational in nature. Basically, if there's no indication that the study participants were asked to do something different about their diet or lifestyle, the study was probably observational.

In the chapters that follow, we'll be looking at some classic examples of observational studies, including the Seven Countries Study and the Framingham Heart Study.

Controlled Trials

Controlled trials are where the whole "cause and effect" thing starts to become decipherable. This form of research involves taking at least two groups of participants, including a control group and one or more experimental groups, in order to gauge the effect of a particular treatment. The control group is deliberately excluded from the variable or variables being tested, while the experimental group gets exposed to some sort of change—like a new diet, medication, or exercise program. When compared with the control group, the results of the experimental group make it possible to gauge the effects of that change, without the infamous confounding that happens in observational studies.

But not all controlled trials are created equal. The gold standard of controlled research is the randomized controlled trial (RCT)—where participants aren't only assigned to control or experimental groups, but are also randomized, meaning they're placed into those groups by chance rather than choice. That weeds out the bias that happens when people choose for themselves which group they want to be in. (RCTs can be cranked up an even higher notch when they're double-blind, where the participants aren't told which group they ended up in, and the investigators don't know either. That way, nobody's power of expectation can influence the study's outcome or the interpretation of its results.)

A lot of controlled trials will specify the level of prevention they're targeting, including the following:

Primary prevention aims to prevent a disease before it ever happens—in other words, to keep healthy people healthy.

Secondary prevention aims to slow or halt a disease after it's already been diagnosed (or after serious risk factors for the disease have popped up).

Tertiary prevention aims to help folks manage complicated health problems after they've already taken root—like full-fledged heart disease, cancer, and diabetes.

Systematic Reviews and Meta-Analyses

Many researchers consider systematic reviews and meta-analyses to be the shining stars of important research, and in some ways, that's often the case. *Systematic reviews* focus on a specific question and attempt to answer it with the best available research literature.

In addition to combining data from various studies, *meta-analyses* also contrast the results. The goal is to gauge the overall direction of the evidence, accounting for outliers and identifying patterns that might not emerge when looking at each study individually.

Both these forms of research help us gain a more global perspective of a particular issue and catapult our understanding to new heights.

On the flip side, both systematic reviews and meta-analyses are only as strong as the evidence they draw from (and the criteria investigators use when choosing which studies to incorporate).

How to Read a Scientific Paper

First and foremost, do *not* read a scientific paper from top to bottom, title to references, like you would a novel or magazine article, unless you truly enjoy gratuitous pain. Your job is to be a sleuth, not a masochist. And if you're after the meat of the paper instead of the fluffy trimmings, there's plenty you can skip over while still getting the gist. Focus on getting in, out, and on with life. Luckily, scientific papers share some basic anatomy that we can break down for the sake of easy digestibility. Let's dissect.

The Abstract is a summary that sits at the top of the paper under the title and author information. This is supposed to be the *CliffsNotes* version of the research at hand—a recap of what the study was about, what it found, and what those findings mean. It can be tempting to just read the abstract and stop there, assuming you already know the most important parts of the paper. But that's the worst possible thing you can do. This leads to the debilitating condition *abstractitis*, which runs rampant among people who want to win arguments they do not fully understand.

The abstract should serve as a screening device only—something to help us weed out rat experiments when we're looking for human trials, or studies on alcohol when we're researching caffeine. Abstracts work as a rough gauge to tell us whether or not the rest of the paper is worth reading. But keep in mind that the abstract is only a reflection of the authors' interpretation of their own work—and that may or may not reveal the full picture. As a health sleuth, your mission, if you choose to accept it, is to read on.

The Introduction relays what the findings of previous research on the subject, what knowledge gaps still exist, and what the author's (or authors') objectives were for the study.

The Materials and Methods section describes the study's design, how it was executed, and who participated in it. This section and the *Results* section are the most important sections of any paper. These are the *only* safe zones in the paper that, for the most part, stay unmarred by any biases or preconceptions the authors might drag with them into the study. From these two sections alone, you'll be able to tell exactly how the study was conducted and exactly what it found.

The Results section unveils the cold, hard data the study churned up—often accompanied by graphs, charts, tables, and other visuals to intrigue and bedazzle you. It's a good idea to read the Results section *before* looking at the author's interpretation of what he or she found. Even if you have a will of steel, it's hard to avoid being swayed by another's view of the data. Before the paper has a chance to brainwash you, ask yourself: what does the data *say?* The Results section is like the spec sheet on a car purchase—the straight dope before salespeople get a chance to razzle-dazzle you with their own spin on things. While reading through this section, you might need to pause and jump into the *Methods* section to make sense of what's going on. That's perfectly all right.

The Discussion section is the author's interpretation of his or her findings, explaining any strengths or shortcomings of the study. Here is where you really need to put on your sleuthing cap. If the author or authors did drag any biases or preconceived notions into the study, the Discussion section is where they'll bloom like weeds. Remember, the reason we want to read a scientific paper instead of rely on other people's summaries of it is to *check for validity.* We want to see what the researcher did, what was found, and whether the conclusions are justified. Believe it or not, you don't always need a deep background in biostats. You just need to ask a few questions as you read this section. These might include:

Are there any trends in the data that the authors didn't point out?

Are the authors trying to squeeze anomalous findings into the mold of conventional wisdom? (For example: are they emphasizing short-comings of their study design to explain why their research didn't find what they'd expected?)

Are the researchers funded by, or associated with, any companies or agencies that would have a vested interest in the outcome of the study?

The References list corresponds to footnotes in the article. Whenever you spot one of those little numbers perched after a phrase or sentence, it means the authors are using another study or paper to back up a claim they've made, and you can track it down yourself in the reference list.

Now that we've explored some basics of research and how to decipher it, let's talk about something more delicious: fat!

6
Reopening the Case Against Saturated Fat

OUT OF ALL THE FOOD PYRAMID'S VICTIMS, the most brutally slaughtered was *fat*—particularly the saturated form. Stuffed into the use-sparingly tip alongside sugar, fat became immortalized as a wasteland of empty calories, appropriate only for a rare and guilt-laden indulgence. Even the pyramid's 2011 upgrade, the circular MyPlate, continues the ultra-lean legacy: nowhere is the existence of fat even acknowledged.

While attitudes about fat are beginning to change—evidenced by the ever-growing selection of olive oils available at the supermarket— *saturated* fat still remains firmly blacklisted. Its image as a thief of health is so widespread, in fact, that we rarely stop and question what crimes it actually committed—or, for that matter, examine the evidence that handed down the guilty verdict in the first place. The term "saturated fat" is virtually wed to its descriptor "artery clogging," reinforcing the thought of a deadly (albeit delicious) substance sludging through our veins like grease through a pipe. Each bite supposedly lands us a little closer to a heart attack. And it works its black magic, we're told, through an equally frightful avenue: cholesterol in our blood.

It might come as a surprise, then, that the case against saturated fat was never a foregone conclusion. Rather, it was cobbled together with pieces of observational data, short-term trials, animal studies, and guesswork, resulting in a theory that—even today—generates paradoxes and contradictions rather than adequately explaining the state of human health.

In this chapter, we'll trace the evolution of the nation's grudge against fat (and its partner in crime, cholesterol), and explore how its saturated form shifted from nourishment to nemesis. We'll learn about two of the nutrition world's most game-changing postulates—the lipid hypothesis and diet-heart hypothesis—as well as the studies and masterminds that ushered them into being. It's a saga that starts in the arteries of some unfortunate bunnies and ends in a battlefield of bad science.

The Lipid Hypothesis

In 1913, Russian researcher Nikolai Anichkov sealed one of the first links in the chain that bound cholesterol to heart disease—a connection that would later lure fat into a federal food fight that continues to rage today. Like other scientists of his time, Anichkov had been sleuthing out the cause of *atherosclerosis,* a term dubbed in 1904 to describe the mysterious, waxy plaque accumulation found on the walls of arteries.[1]

It was a time when rabbit studies were en vogue, and one of Anichkov's contemporaries, Russian scientist Alexander Ignatovski, managed to induce plaque in the arteries of rabbits by swapping their vegetarian diet with a more carnivorous meat-and-egg-based menu. Yet neither Ignatovski nor other researchers had figured out *what* in the carnivore diet, exactly, caused arteries to fill with plaque. (Many suspected it might be protein, believed at the time to accelerate the aging process.[2])

Anichkov famously solved the mystery. Through a series of progressively honed experiments, feeding rabbits various foods and then their isolated components, he pinpointed dietary cholesterol (or *cholesterin,* as it was called back then) as the culprit. For the first time, he showed that feeding rabbits pure cholesterol was enough to induce atherosclerosis similar to that found in humans. His early studies, for the record, employed diets with 5 percent cholesterol by weight—the equivalent of a human gorging on about a hundred eggs per day.[3]

But here's the interesting thing: Anichkov was never fully convinced that the results of his rabbit studies translated to humans. For one, rabbits, unlike humans, are hardcore herbivores—equipped with labyrinth-like digestive systems, a fondness for all things fiber, and a complete lack of predatory skills. So it's no real surprise that stuffing them with foods foreign to their species would create unfavorable results. They don't have the anatomy to digest cholesterol any more than we humans have the anatomy to digest nylon stockings or BB pellets.

So Anichkov and his colleagues, to clarify the effects of cholesterol on different creatures, conducted similar experiments using rats and guinea pigs—only to discover that the same dietary cholesterol that injured the arteries of one species often did nada to another.

With conflicting evidence at his fingertips, Anichkov cautioned against jumping to conclusions about whether dietary cholesterol was a threat for humans. In a 1913 paper titled, "On experimental cholesterin steatosis and its significance in the origin of some pathological processes," he explained it as follows:

> On the basis of the rat experiments described above, we conclude that the harmful effect of cholesterin-rich nourishment is not expressed equally in all types of animals…. The fact that cholesterin has different effects on different animals, even closely related ones, raises the question as to what degree the results described above are valid for human pathology.[4]

Indeed, if you'll recall from our *Hitchhiker's Guide* chapter, one of the caveats with animal studies is the difference—often vast—between humans and critters, particularly when it comes to physiology and metabolism. Just as one man's trash is another man's treasure, one species' poison may be another's healthy breakfast. Animal models, whether rabbit or rat or housefly, are best used to tweeze apart biological processes, pinpoint the roles of various genes, and help shape the direction of more sophisticated human studies. But when it comes to how we should fuel our bodies, they offer little to no real guidance.

From that perspective, Anichkov's studies showed pretty clearly that rabbits can't handle cholesterol from food: it's promptly dumped into their bloodstream and deposited in unfortunate places around their bodies, including their livers and kidneys and eyelids. But whereas egg-eating rabbits are universally headed toward a future of disease, the same can't be said of egg-eating humans. We might learn more about how that process works by reviewing the case of the eighty-eight-year-old Colorado man, who—after at least fifteen years of eating two-dozen eggs per day—had normal cholesterol levels and zero signs of heart disease.[5] For most humans, the experience would be the same. Although genetic factors can influence how we respond to dietary cholesterol (and do include a good deal of individual variation), the effects, in general, range from minor to naught.

Nonetheless, Anichkov's experiments weren't entirely irrelevant to our two-legged, opposable-thumbed species. They may not have proven anything about the effect of dietary cholesterol on humans, but they did set the framework for a later—more momentous—breakthrough: the role of *blood* cholesterol in heart disease.

The Low-Down on Cholesterol

Before we continue, let's take a quick pit stop at Cholesterol Central to catch our bearings.

Cholesterol is one of those terms we've all heard at some point—whether from a monotone biology teacher or a statin commercial or our own doctor. But most of us have an oversimplified, somewhat cartoonish understanding of the role this substance plays in our bodies, especially when it comes to heart disease.

For starters, the terms "good cholesterol" and "bad cholesterol" are woefully misleading. In reality, there's really only one kind of cholesterol. When we talk about "good cholesterol" and "bad cholesterol," we actually mean *lipoproteins*—high density lipoprotein (HDL) and low density lipoprotein (LDL), respectively—which shuttle cholesterol (and other lipids) around our bodies through the bloodstream. In other words, the stuff we call cholesterol is often referring to cholesterol's *vehicles*—the lipoproteins—rather than the cholesterol itself. Kind of misleading, right?

And rather than your body's perverted attempt to convert its innards into a self-made poison, cholesterol is actually quite a rock star substance. It's crucial for synthesizing vitamin D and sex hormones like estrogen and testosterone, building cell membranes, and making bile acids to help you digest food. If you somehow managed to eradicate cholesterol from your body, you would be very much dead.

Where the problem comes in is when your body's fabulous balance of cholesterol transportation and cleanup goes awry. Think of LDL particles as taxis—driving little cholesterol passengers out from your liver to wherever it is they need to go in the body. Your cells have LDL receptors to pull those particles in and unload the cholesterol.

By contrast, HDL comes along dump-truck style and whisks excess cholesterol away, returning it to the liver for your body to recycle or eliminate. (Maybe that's not the nicest way to treat former taxi passengers, but frankly, your body is a pretty brutal place to live.)

Now imagine what happens when those LDL taxis get stuck in traffic and spend ages driving around in your bloodstream. We'd end up with some cranky cholesterol passengers, right? Just like cars on a congested highway, LDL particles can spend far too long circulating in your blood, becoming unruly road-rage terrors as a result.

This basically describes the process known as *oxidation*. You see, when cholesterol leaves your liver, it's packaged with some helpful antioxidant goodies to sustain it for the journey, as well as protect it from reacting with unstable molecules hanging out in your blood.

But once the store of antioxidants are depleted, all bets are off: the LDL becomes subject to damage and attack, leading to molecular changes that render it invisible to the LDL receptors that usually reel it in. What's more, once LDL oxidizes, your body sees it as a foreign invader, and unleashes its immune-system army to wage war. And that sets off a cascade of other processes ultimately leading to what we know as atherosclerotic heart disease.

Although there's a host of additional steps involved in plaque buildup and heart attacks, for now, it's just worth noting that LDL becomes the biggest threat when it gets oxidized (or damaged in other ways, including through the effects of infection). Ultimately, high levels of LDL are a problem insofar as more LDL means more "traffic" and slower clearance from your blood, both of which increase its risk of oxidation.

So what turns your bloodstream into the LDL equivalent of Seattle's rush hour? As we'll see in the next chapter, saturated fat often gets the blame due to its cholesterol-raising abilities: it tends to reduce the activity of your LDL receptors, allowing more LDL particles to swim through your bloodstream at once—though the extent of that varies from person to person and depends on the type of saturated fat consumed. (Saturated fat also bestows other qualities that actually reduce LDL oxidation, too, so its effect may be a wash in some sense.)

Obesity, smoking, sedentary living, stress, and certain diseases and drugs can also increase circulating LDL levels. And apart from that, some conditions like familial hypercholesterolemia—a genetic defect that slashes LDL receptor activity—can cause cholesterol levels to sky-rocket well beyond what most people could normally achieve, with extreme LDL oxidation and early heart disease often on its heels.

What's more, contrary to the portrayal most of us are familiar with, our arteries *aren't* some sort of simple plumbing system, subject to gumming up with all that cholesterol floating around. And the solution isn't a massive Roto-Rooter in the form of a quadruple bypass to scrape it all out, either. Quite the contrary!

Arterial plaque actually builds up *beneath* the walls of your arteries, and is full of calcium, bloated immune cells, and oxidized LDL. If you're curious about the full story of arterial plaque and how heart disease develops, check out Chris Masterjohn's website *The Daily Lipid* (http://blog.cholesterol-and-health.com/). He offers one of the most integrative and intelligent explanations of cholesterol's role in heart disease that I have thus far encountered.

Now, as you read on, bear in mind that the earliest forays into heart disease research didn't have the luxury of our current cholesterol knowledge. Total cholesterol—without distinguishing between different types of lipoproteins or the oxidation process—was typically the only measurement available or understood. Heart disease, while still imperfectly grasped today, was even more of a mystery back then. The discovery process very much launched from intellectual scratch. So it's hard to judge our early heart disease trailblazers for not knowing what we know today.

That's Not All, Folks

Let's now return briefly to our Russian scientist, Anichkov. Differences between bunny and man aside, his research gave the world of science the *lipid hypothesis,* which states that deranged blood lipids—particularly elevated cholesterol—play a central role in heart disease.

It wasn't until the 1970s that the term lipid hypothesis appeared verbatim in any literature. But once it did, it began to drive the mammoth industry of statin drugs, various interventions to reduce cholesterol levels, and even the cost of your life insurance.

Bear in mind that the lipid hypothesis, per its true definition, concerns itself only with the makeup of the blood. It *doesn't* directly comment on what factors—for example, diet, smoking, stress levels, and exercise (or lack thereof)—drive those blood lipids into disarray. This is the clear distinction between the lipid hypothesis and the diet-heart hypothesis that we'll expand on shortly.

And despite the eventual clout that Anichkov's hypothesis gained, it lay dormant for decades—lost as an unconnected dot in the heart disease saga until one man brought it back to the fore: a researcher named Ancel Keys.

7
Ancel Keys and the Diet-Heart Hypothesis

ONCE IN A GREAT WHILE a figure emerges boldly from the abyss and spends eternity saddled with equal parts love and hate, prestige and controversy, reverence and angst. AT&T commercials had their Carrot Top. Seinfeld had its Newman. And the world of nutrition had a man named Ancel Keys.

Keys—or "Monsieur Cholesterol," as a Belgian maître d' once dubbed him—entered the nutrition scene from humble beginnings. Born to teenage parents in Colorado, Keys spent his youth as a lumber camp worker, a powder monkey in a goldmine, and a bat guano shoveler in an Arizonan cave—with later jaunts landing him as a clerk in a Woolworth store and an oiler aboard the China-bound *S.S. President Wilson,* where he endured his first dietary experiment: living on almost nothing but alcohol.[1] But none of those experiences, however titillating, could compare with the work Keys would later do in the field of health.

After racking up degrees in political science, biology, oceanography, and physiology in his characteristically diverse fashion, Keys launched his legacy as a researcher. By the 1940s, he'd shown the world his nutrition chops when he developed the legendary K-ration meal for soldiers in combat. (The K stands for Keys.) Though the ready-made meals—small enough to fit in a cargo pocket and containing canned meat chunks, hard biscuits, and malted milk tablets—averaged a rating of "better than nothing" when soldiers were polled for their gustatory opinion, the K-ration became an infantry mainstay, with more than 105 million produced in 1944 alone.[2]

The Minnesota Starvation Experiment

After earning his nutrition stripes with the K-rations, Keys led the Minnesota Starvation Experiment—a groundbreaking study that defined our modern understanding of food deprivation and weight loss. Unfortunately, the study's grim message has been lost amid today's modern diet culture.

In a trial that might seem a bit horrifying by today's standards, Keys and his colleagues recruited thirty-six young, healthy, conscientious objectors to the war—all to be systematically starved in the name of science. For six months starting in November of 1944, the volunteers eked by on half of their normal calorie needs. Their two-meals-per-day diet was designed to mimic the sparse, starchy diet of war-ravaged Europe, consisting of little more than rutabagas, potatoes, cabbage, and bread. By the end of those six stomach-growling months, the men had lost a full quarter of their original body weight and nearly all of their mental bearings.

The study wasn't a matter of cruel and unusual punishment, but an attempt to brace for the war's eventual aftermath. The Minnesota experiment sent out probes into the then-dark landscape of starvation—both to learn how extreme hunger would impact the body and mind, and to determine how war-torn countries could best rehabilitate their famished survivors after the close of combat.

The results were profound: not only did food deprivation lead to weight loss and physical discomfort, but also to nightmarish psychological shifts. As their bodies eroded further and further toward emaciation, the study's volunteers found themselves spiraling into the depths of depression, hypochondria, obsession, and even compulsive self-mutilation. Across the board, the men's libidos vanished. Physical strength dwindled to frailty. Thoughts of food seized every waking moment. Some men, in fact, took to collecting dozens of cookbooks as if they were thriller novels. Others shoplifted vegetables and binged on them. And still others developed strange fascinations with watching other people eat.

To the surprise of all, the refeeding process proved even more brutal than starvation itself. Once the men—whittled to a shadow of their formers selves—were allowed to gradually increase their food intake, psychological neuroses reared even more dramatically. One participant sliced off three of his own fingers with an ax, lost in such a cognitive haze that he couldn't tell whether he'd done it on purpose or by accident.[3]

In some cases, the men's altruism and desire to serve humanity—those very qualities that brought them to conscientious war objection in the first place—weakened along with their bodies, replaced by disinterest in the outside world and total fixation on food. By September 1945, Japan's war-ending surrender barely fazed the men, who'd been eating dinner when the announcement came. "The food was the important thing," said study participant Jay Garner, whose frame dwindled from 165 pounds to 119 during the course of the experiment. "We didn't care whether the war was over or not as long as we got our food."[4]

Although the study ended too late to benefit postwar relief efforts, its findings have shed invaluable light on the physiology and psychology of eating disorders, and other situations of energy deprivation. From this seminal work, we now know that anorexia, for instance, can be a *result* of malnutrition rather than its initial cause. (The complete findings were published in a book titled *The Biology of Human Starvation*, a two-volume, still-cherished gem among psychologists and physiologists.)

With science's ethical standards facing a post-war revolution, largely due to the horror rippling across the globe when knowledge of Nazi experiments surfaced, it may have been the last time in history that starvation could be used to conduct a nutrition study. The effects of deprivation were not lost on Keys, either.

"Starved people cannot be taught democracy," he declared after the war, in an apt merging of both his political science and physiology backgrounds. "To talk about the will of the people when you aren't feeding them is perfect hogwash."[5]

In today's weight-loss-obsessed world, the findings of the Minnesota Starvation Experiment cannot be overstated—making their obscurity in the mainstream all the more troubling. The men's physical and mental turmoil emerged on diets averaging 1,500 to 1,600 calories per day, plus consistent physical activity—levels well within the range of many crash-diet fads plenty of us follow today.

More important, though, the study shows what can happen when we deliberately and severely eat less than our body is asking for.

Think about that for a minute. The same health authorities propagating food-pyramid wisdom also tend to fixate on cutting calories and increasing exercise—the "eat less, move more" paradigm. Sounds familiar, doesn't it?

Now think about the hyper-palatable, low-satiation foods dominating the American menu. They may be the very reason our "full" signals have gone AWOL, leaving our hands scraping the bottom of the Doritos bag long after we should have stopped eating. What if calorie restricting makes our bodies think we're starving? And what if what happened to the Minnesota men at 1,500 calories is what our government and the billion dollar diet industry has been selling to modern Westerners? The answer seems clear enough: we've set ourselves up to be a nation of disordered eaters, struggling against biology, when what really needs to change is the quality of our food.

Cholesterol: The First Strike of the Inning

It wasn't until after the war—and the fascinating conclusion of his starvation study—that Keys stepped on the path that would not only put his name on the map, but also land his face on the cover of *Time* magazine. As the dust from combat settled and death statistics emerged in its wake, Keys noticed something peculiar: heart disease mortality had dropped rapidly in zones where food rationing had been in place—while elsewhere in the industrialized world, including in the obituary column of his local newspaper, death from heart disease seemed to be skyrocketing. And men, it appeared, were the illness's chief victims.

Intrigued by the seemingly connectable dots, Keys embarked on the first of his diet-heart adventures: a study of about three hundred middle-aged businessmen from Minnesota, whose lives would soon become precious data points for science. Falling under the umbrella of a *prospective cohort* design, the study followed the men for the next fifteen years, watching hawkishly for any traits separating those who developed heart disease from those who were spared. It was a hunt for what would later be coined "risk factors"—that is, variables associated with disease incidence, such as smoking or stress.

It didn't take long before one particular blood marker blew the rest of the risk factors out of the water: *total* cholesterol. The research found that the higher the men's total cholesterol level, the more likely they were to perish from heart disease as the years rolled on—a trend that also materialized in other observational studies across the country.

So the same waxy substance hijacking the arteries of Anichkov's rabbits was suddenly back in the spotlight, this time surging through the blood of humans. Keys described it with unflinching detail: "The cholesterol gets deposited in the arteries until it looks as if someone has dumped Cream of Wheat in them."[6] (As fat increasingly appeared to be standing on the wrong end of a smoking gun, that imagery shifted from hot cereal toward descriptions of greasy, fatty sludge.)

Though compelling, the study was far from perfect, because the subjects were all the same age, gender, and socioeconomic status, and shared similar lifestyles. (And, as it later turned out, the same group for whom blood cholesterol best predicts heart disease— middle-aged men with stressful jobs—just so happened to be the same folks Keys recruited into his study.) It'd take a few somersaults of logic to generalize the study's findings to more diverse populations. Still, the new lead was enough to set Keys hot on heart disease's trail. Only one question remained: what caused cholesterol to rise?

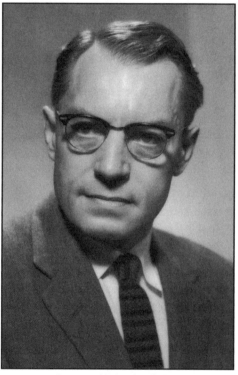

Courtesy of University of Minnesota Archives

Fig. 8. Nutrition Scientist Ancel Keys

Six Countries and a Hypothesis

By 1953, Ancel Keys had drawn the first pen stroke in what would become a long, intricate game of hangman for saturated fat. Using food intake data and mortality statistics from the late 1940s, he created a simple but compelling graph. For six countries—Japan, Italy,

Six Countries or Seven? One of the most common misinterpretations of Ancel Keys's career involves his Six Country Analysis and his Seven Countries Study—sometimes thought to be one and the same, no doubt due to their similar names. However, these projects were two very different things: the Six Countries Analysis was a simple graph plotting fat intake against national heart disease mortality, which Keys carefully penned in the early 1950s; the Seven Countries Study was a massive *prospective cohort* project launched at the end of the same decade and that's still—over half a century later—churning out new waves of analyses.

England, Australia, Canada, and the USA—he plotted national fat intake against each country's rate of death from heart disease. The result was a nearly perfect upward curve: the more fat a country's citizens ate, the more heart disease that country faced—a prime opportunity for mistaking *correlation for causation* if there ever was one. Unfortunately, reality proved to be bit more complicated.

Although somewhat crude by today's standards, the graph seemed momentous at the time—and it kick-started Keys's career-long habit of stretching population data in directions it couldn't comfortably reach. Armed with the conviction that fat was responsible for heart disease, Keys went public with his theory and set out to inform the world.

What Keys was chasing—and would remain in hot pursuit of for the rest of his career—is what we now call the *diet-heart hypothesis,* or the idea that saturated fat ("diet") causes cardiovascular disease ("heart" disease) by raising blood cholesterol. It basically piggybacks off Anichkov's lipid hypothesis, adding one more link to the chain by claiming that saturated fat is the culprit behind those heart-disease-inducing hikes in cholesterol. It's a concept that would spend decades tumbling around a sea of skepticism before docking amid scientific consensus, due in no small part to Keys navigating it there.

In 1955, Keys presented his Six Countries curve at the World Health Organization (WHO) conference in Geneva, amid a gathering of great and forward-thinking minds. Drawing from a range of animal studies, population data, blood cholesterol trends, and other evidence he'd carefully knitted together, Keys explained his graph and theory with unflappable confidence and waited for awe to sweep over the audience.[7]

DIET-HEART HYPOTHESIS VS. LIPID HYPOTHESIS

While the lipid hypothesis states only that blood lipids, particularly elevated cholesterol, play a central role in heart disease, the argument for the diet-heart hypothesis zeros in on **saturated fat** as the culprit. The logic goes like this: high blood cholesterol causes heart disease, and saturated fat raises blood cholesterol, so saturated fat must raise heart disease risk.

With that in mind, we can sum up the difference between these two hypotheses as follows:

Lipid hypothesis: high cholesterol in the blood causes heart disease.

Diet-heart hypothesis: high saturated fat intake causes high cholesterol in the blood, which causes heart disease.

Technically speaking, theories about cholesterol oxidation, HDL to total cholesterol ratio, lipoprotein particle size, and other lipid-related issues also fall under the lipid hypothesis's umbrella.

But here's where the two hypotheses get confusing: because it's so widely accepted by mainstream medicine that saturated fat hikes up blood cholesterol, the diet-heart hypothesis and the lipid hypothesis are sometimes used interchangeably—with the former having absorbed the latter in the minds of many scientists and other health authorities.

It's important to view the two as separate entities, though, especially as we plow deeper into the scientific expeditions of the last century. Researcher Daniel Steinberg emphasized the need for this distinction in his book *The Cholesterol Wars: The Skeptics vs. The Preponderance of Evidence*.

The fact is, cholesterol and other lipids in the blood can cause heart disease without the presence of saturated fat. What's more, the diet-heart hypothesis rests on surprisingly weak evidence—something we'll explore further in the coming pages. But even as we knock down the diet-heart hypothesis, bear in mind that its shortcomings don't necessarily invalidate the lipid hypothesis. Conflating the two only muddies the already murky waters of heart disease research.

To Keys's surprise, his presentation was met with more ridicule than respect. Sir George Pickering, a physician and college head at Oxford, baited him with the question, "If you would be so kind, Professor Keys, what do you consider the single best piece of evidence to support your diet-heart idea?"[8]

No match for the debate-savvy Brit, Keys didn't realize he'd been lured into a rhetorical trap. And his mistake? Instead of supplying a body of evidence from multiple sources, Keys relied on a *single* piece of evidence: his graph. And unable to summon his usually quick wit, he fumbled in his response to Pickering. The move proved to be a disastrous one. Fellow WHO attendants, eager to play Keys for a fool, promptly dismissed the graph and silenced any further attempt to claim fat as the cause of heart disease. A crestfallen Keys returned to America with no more allies than when he'd left.

The aftermath of the WHO conference didn't end when he set foot on the soil of his own country, either. In another blow, Berkeley statistician Jacob Yerushalmy and New York State Commissioner of Health Herman Hilleboe—who both attended the WHO meeting with Keys—whipped up a scathing critique of the Six-Country graph. In their 1957 paper "Fat in the diet and mortality from heart disease: a methodological note," the men exposed cracks in Keys's logic in a way only the savviest of number-crunchers can do.[9]

The paper opened with an almost clairvoyant exposé of traps that would plague epidemiology for decades to come: Yerushalmy and Hilleboe emphasized that observational associations could never prove cause and effect (remember our lesson from *Hitchhiker's Guide?*) and warned that other factors often obscure the relationship between things that seem to march in step, side by side. "It is always necessary to probe further, to go beyond the simple, apparent association and to investigate related variables," they wrote.

Continuing, Yerushalmy and Hilleboe pointed out that Keys's Six-Country graph had turned into something of a fish story—growing bigger and more impressive with each retelling, like a guppy morphing into Moby Dick after some exaggeration (and maybe a few too many beers) on the part of its fisherman. When Keys first described the graph in a 1953 paper, he'd been careful with his phrasing, stating only: "It must be concluded that dietary fat somehow is associated with cardiac disease mortality, at least in middle age."

By 1954, the graph became a bit mightier through the words of another researcher, who wrote in a *Lancet* paper: "There appears to be a strong if not convincing correlation between the amount of fat in the diet and the death rate from degenerative heart disease." And a year later, the guppy-like graph had bloomed into a majestic white whale: Keys abandoned his previous restraint, calling the correlation between fat and heart disease "remarkable" and adding that "no other variable in the mode of life besides the fat calories [shows] such a consistent relationship to the mortality rate from coronary or degenerative heart disease."

Somehow, Keys maneuvered his graph into the realm of "damning evidence" in the span of just three years—an impressive feat for six dots on a page. And it wasn't because a calculator-wielding god had descended from the heavens and granted it the power of proving cause and effect, either. The problem was one Yerushalmy and Hilleboe were all too aware of, and one that continues to pollute science more than half a century later: associations can seem like certainties if they're repeated often enough. They wrote,

> Quotation and repetition of the suggestive association soon creates the impression that the relationship is truly valid, and ultimately it acquires status as a supporting link in a chain of presumed proof.

And that's not all Yerushalmy and Hilleboe had to say. They questioned Keys's methodology and whether he had *really* scoured all the data. Keys had graphed only six countries when Yerushalmy and Hilleboe discovered data for twenty-two had been available. Keys acknowledged this issue in his 1953 paper—stating that Western Germany and Finland were unreliable due to postwar population shifts; Iceland and Luxembourg didn't have enough citizens to yield reliable data; and Spain lacked vital statistics in the late 1940s—but he remained vague about what was wrong with all the other nations booted from his analysis. Keys simply wrote, "So far it has been possible to get fully comparable dietary and vital statistics data from six countries," never explaining what his criteria for "fully comparable" actually included.

The fact that the six countries that *did* make the cut—Japan, Italy, England and Wales, Australia, Canada, and the USA—were the exact ones needed to form a flawless upward curve on a graph has led to much eyebrow raising, especially among critics who question Keys's vague selection strategy.

To paint a more complete picture, Yerushalmy and Hilleboe took the data for *all* available countries, plotting each nation's average fat intake with its rate of heart disease in men—much in the same way Keys had done. (See Table 1.)

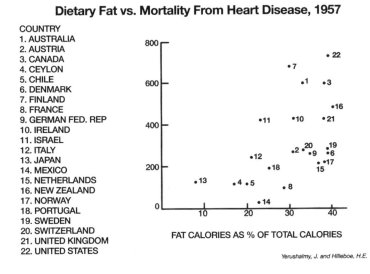

TABLE 1. A representation of Yerushalmy and Hilleboe's chart detailing mortality from heart disease (arteriosclerotic and degenerative) and percent of calories from dietary fat in 22 countries: men, aged 55-59, 1950.

They found *some* sort of relationship between saturated fat and heart disease—one that remained "statistically significant" in math-speak, meaning it probably wasn't due to random chance. But the loose splattering of dots was much less compelling than Keys's eerily perfect curve. For instance, France and Finland had virtually identical intakes of fat, yet Finland suffered from heart disease at rates seven times greater. Yerushalmy and Hilleboe remarked that even though a positive relationship seemed to exist, Keys's graph had "greatly exaggerated the importance of the association." Clearly fat wasn't the only heart-harming force at play, if it was even directly responsible at all.

Yerushalmy and Hilleboe also dug up data for all the macronutrient variables available—testing Keys's claim that nothing was more consistently linked to heart disease mortality than "calories from fat."

After crunching the numbers for each nation's intake of calories, animal fat, animal protein, vegetable fat, vegetable protein, total protein, and carbohydrate, the two researchers emerged with a far different picture than Keys had painted. They found fat and protein derived from animals, *as well as total calorie intake*, bore the strongest correlation with heart disease—not just total fat. The "total fat" Keys focused on for his 1953 graph was essentially a reflection of national meat and dairy consumption.

Although their findings on saturated fat and protein might sound like the death knell for omnivores, Yerushalmy and Hilleboe didn't suggest the world go vegan. Instead, they posed a new question: how did fat—and by extension, animal products—relate to *other* causes of death? After all, heart disease is not the only way to die. Were the folks who were eating more meat and dairy still dropping faster than those who consumed less, once total mortality was considered? The answer came in a compelling table. (See Table 2.)

Correlations between Diet and Death, 1957

Dietary Components †	All Causes of Death	All Causes Other Than Heart Disease	Deaths From Ill-defined or Unknown Causes and Senility
Number of calories			
Total calories	-0.189	-0.580	-0.549
Calories from fat	-0.340	-0.674	-0.453
Animal fat (N = 21)**	-0.169	-0.466	-0.592
Vegetable fat (N = 22) **	-0.339	0.296	0.461
Calories from protein	-0.067	-0.398	-0.487
Animal protein	-0.099	-0.505	-0.572
Vegetable protein	0.275	0.452	0.200
Calories from carbohydrate	0.204	0.172	-0.469
Percent of total calories			
From fat	-0.372	-0.657	-0.375
Animal fat (N = 21)**	-0.178	-0.481	-0.592
Vegetable fat (N = 22)**	-0.277	-0.090	0.632
From protein	0.235	-0.086	-0.275
Animal protein	-0.106	-0.405	-0.479
Vegetable protein	0.187	0.521	0.442
From carbohydrate	0.396	0.671	0.352

* Males 55 to 59 years.
† Calculated from national food balance data by F.A.O.(see text for definition)
** Data not available in France

TABLE 2. A representation of Yerushalmy and Hilleboe's chart correlating the components of diet and death from all causes, from causes other than heart disease, and from ill-defined or unknown causes and senility: men, aged 55-59.

Take another good look at those graphs in Tables 1 and 2.

Now let's translate. Remember, a minus sign in front of a correlation means the association is *negative*. As one variable goes up, the other goes down—a bit like how the higher the temperature outside, the less clothing you're probably sporting. So we can see that when it comes to death from *any* cause—the scroll of values in that first column—fat was not only vindicated, but perhaps also given a back-pat for a job well done on the longevity front. Calories from fat now had the strongest *negative* association with mortality out of any variable, an *r-value* of -0.37. That means the more dietary fat that people consumed, the longer they generally lived. Yerushalmy and Hilleboe found the pattern repeated with animal fat and animal protein, too.

The trend was clear: nations with higher animal fat intake seem to live longer than those with more plant-dominant menus. (If we hop over to that second column—death from non-heart-related causes—we see the same trend holds true to an even more striking degree: animal fat and protein variables are strongly, inversely associated with non-cardiac deaths, while plant-based food variables are positively or neutrally associated.)

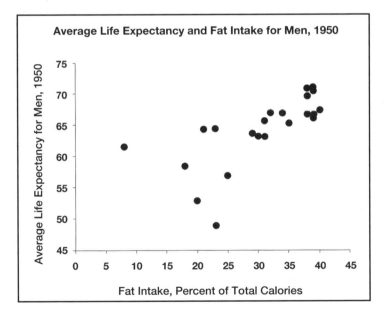

TABLE 3. According to data collected by Yerushalmy and Hilleboe, nations with higher fat intake in 1950 seemed to be living longer than those with lower fat menus. Data source from Earth Trends (http://earthtrends.wri.org/).

To better illustrate this, I've graphed the life expectancy for these same countries in 1950 against their fat intake. (See Table 3.) Although the dots are pretty scattered when fat is below 25 percent of calories, the trend becomes clear once the intake hits the 30 percent mark: *countries with higher average fat intake had the longest life expectancies.*

But did any of this—the life expectancy graph or Yerushalmy and Hilleboe's table of correlations—prove that eating more animal-derived fat and protein was *making* people live longer? Or that eating more carbohydrates and plant foods were *making* them die sooner? Certainly not.

Once again, Yerushalmy and Hilleboe refrained from making any hasty generalizations from those findings. Like a Tootsie Pop, the data had a few more licks to go before reaching its gooey center. Explaining why it'd be a bad idea to interpret a cause-and-effect relationship from anything they'd written so far, the men noted:

> ... fat calories and animal protein calories, which were seen ... to be positively associated with heart disease, are here negatively associated with noncardiac diseases. [A] plausible explanation is that the dietary components which according to the rank correlation coefficients appeared to be positively related to heart disease are indices which reflect attributes of the various countries. That is, it may be that the amount of fat and protein available for consumption is an index of a country's development, industrially, nutritionally, medically, and no doubt in other respects as well.

In other words, animal fat and protein were proxies for a country's overall development, perhaps more than any other component of diet. So what Keys had stumbled upon—and what Yerushalmy and Hilleboe had further illuminated—was that fat intake was a reflection of meat and dairy consumption. But meat and dairy consumption, in turn, were surrogate markers for a nation's wealth. The more of those foods a country managed to stock inside its borders, the more affluent the country was likely to be—in the same way a Mercedes parked in a garage might indicate that household's annual salary.

So what if we plot fat intake against each nation's gross domestic product (GDP) per capita? Take a look at Table 4, and you'll notice that the relationship between diet and national wealth becomes pretty

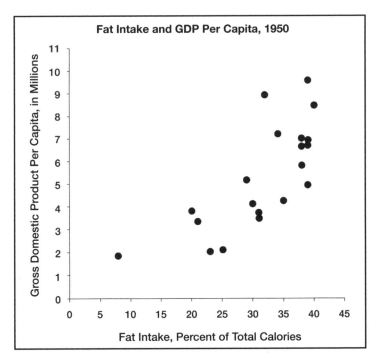

TABLE 4. Data compiled in the 1950s by Yerushalmy and Hilleboe shows that the amount of fat and protein available for consumption in a country correlates with that country's development, suggesting that other trappings of affluence besides dietary fat should be investigated as potential contributing factors in heart disease.

darn clear. (The GDP per capita, or the measure of a country's economic output divided by its population, is a good way to estimate standard of living.[10]) Remember this chart and Yerushalmy and Hilleboe's research as we explore later in the chapter other factors of modern-day affluence.

The problem, of course, is that if meat and saturated fat go hand-in-hand with affluence, they also get tangled up with other features of wealth and industrialization that could damage heart health. That makes the relationship between diet and disease difficult, if not impossible, to decipher from crude correlations.

If that's not enough, consider this: the dietary data from those twenty-two countries—as well as the subset of six that Keys had used—came from balance sheets produced by the Food and Agriculture Organization (FAO), which showed how much food was *available* for consumption in each country, not necessarily how much food was actually consumed. If that sounds like a bizarre and unreliable way to measure what people actually ate, indeed it is. Yerushalmy and Hilleboe explain:

These indices [of food availability] were constructed … from statistics on production, imports, exports, and on the proportion of available food used for purposes other than human nutrition. The underlying data are stated by FAO to be subject to great limitations. Moreover, there are no doubt great differences in food "scraps" in the various countries compared. For example, it is highly probable that far more edible dietary fat is thrown into waste cans in the United States than in less fortunate countries.

And with that came Yerushalmy and Hilleboe's fatal blow to Keys's graph. Not only did national wealth influence how much meat and dairy citizens could access, but it also played a role in how much food never even made it past human lips.

In all, the critique of Keys's work had been devastating—calling into question not just the integrity of his theory, but also his scrupulousness as a researcher. But rather than taking Yerushalmy and Hilleboe's words to heart and acknowledging where he'd flubbed, Keys only fixated harder on his goal.

Fueled by the sting of humiliation from both Geneva and his rival researchers, Keys—no less convinced that fat, in some form or another, was the driving force behind heart disease—became more determined than ever to wipe the bruises from his pride and prove his theory correct. But he wasn't about to repeat the mistakes he'd made in Geneva. In order to shift science's global tides, Keys would need something more compelling. A project that didn't just grab data and sprinkle it on a graph unpolished, but one that employed meticulous methodology. One that was airtight in its analysis. One that lasted long enough to track the development of heart disease in relation to food in a way that silenced all doubts. Keys's dream would soon not only rise into being, but also enter the ranks of science's landmark studies on nutrition—emblazoned under the title of the Seven Countries Study.

The Seven Countries Study

In 1980, when cardiologist Carleton Chapman sat down to pen the foreword to *Seven Countries: A Multivariate Analysis of Death and Coronary Disease,* the task was more than a little bit daunting. "There is no prototype with which to compare Keys's opus," he wrote. "*Seven Countries* in an important sense represents the end of intellectual innocence."[11]

And it was true. The Seven Countries Study was one of those staggering monoliths that permanently altered the landscape of nutrition—built strong enough to withstand even the most destructive of Godzilla-like stompings. In an era where science was just getting warmed up on its heart disease hunt, the study became a milestone, marking the first effort in history to hop international borders and compare diet-disease associations between diverse, culturally unique populations. With the participation of nearly thirteen thousand men aged forty to fifty-nine, the study scoured sixteen regions of seven countries—Greece, Finland, Japan, the Netherlands, Italy, Yugoslavia, and the United States. Today, it remains a pivotal piece of the diet-heart hypothesis that gripped the nation and ultimately public policy.

Although the Seven Countries Study wasn't officially launched until 1958, its conception began seven years earlier in the heart of Italy. In 1951, Keys and his wife Margaret had made their first of what would become many trips to Naples—a visit inspired by its nation's legendary cardiovascular health. "Heart disease is no problem here," an Italian colleague had told Keys. "Come and see for yourself."[12]

As one might imagine, the dangled promise was enough to bait Keys. Never one to stop working, even while on holiday, Keys made it his business to tour Neapolitan hospitals looking for signs of thickened arteries and pain-sieged chests. But the search was fruitless: cardiovascular disease seemed to be a mythical beast in the Italian city—a unicorn of sorts, fabled but unseen. Keys's colleague had been right.

And for Keys, that raised a lot of questions.

What was it about Naples that spared its citizens from heart disease? Were the protective factors there the same as those seen in other healthy-hearted countries? Would any clues about heart disease emerge from cross-cultural comparisons? What did Naples do right that other regions did wrong?

To quench these nagging questions, the Seven Countries Study bloomed into being. Let's now take a look at the findings Keys dredged up, and gauge how we should view this landmark study through the clarity of hindsight.

A Trek in the Dark

As one of the earliest ventures in heart disease epidemiology, the Seven Countries Study began as a guesswork-laden trek through uncharted territory. When the project first kicked off, the plan was to monitor diverse populations and decipher which potential risk factors were truly playing a role in heart disease—with the main contenders of the time being blood pressure, physical activity level, body weight, body mass index, height, smoking habits, resting heart rate, diet, and blood cholesterol. (At the time, scientists hadn't yet clarified the importance of distinguishing different forms of lipoproteins—particularly LDL and HDL—so "total cholesterol" was the only number on their radar.)

Of course, despite its global scope, Seven Countries was bound by the limitations of an observation-only design. As with any study of that ilk, it could only watch from the sidelines while participants tussled with death and disease, accumulating data for investigators to later inspect for patterns. That's where research starts, not where it ends. In his 1980 *Seven Countries* book, Keys even repeated the same type of "correlation doesn't equal causation" lecturing he'd received from Yerushalmy and Hilleboe so many years before, writing (emphasis mine):

> It is interesting to compare characteristics of men given a diagnosis of coronary heart disease with their fellows not so judged, but *conclusions about cause and effect are not warranted from such data.* Many of the characteristics of interest are so interrelated that in single-variable analysis it would be easy to mistake secondary for primary associations.[13]

It was a warning that should come slapped across not only the Seven Countries Study, but also *any* public chunk of epidemiology—in the same way we label flammable substances or electrocution hazards. Its capital, bold letters might read: **THIS STUDY IS SAFE WHEN HANDLED WITH CARE, BUT IT SHOULD NEVER BE ALLOWED TO TRESPASS INTO EVIDENCE TERRITORIES IT DOESN'T RIGHTFULLY BELONG.**

But as we shall very soon see, the Seven Countries Study did just that.

KEYS ON CHOLESTEROL

A little-known fact about Ancel Keys is that he spent his lengthy career believing dietary cholesterol was *not* a threat to heart health. In his 1952 paper "Human atherosclerosis and the diet," he wrote, drawing from animal experiments, "the most reasonable conclusion would be that the cholesterol content of human diets is unimportant in human atherosclerosis."[79] Likewise, in some of his metabolic ward studies, Keys found that altering *dietary cholesterol* had only minor effects on *blood cholesterol*—concluding that "attention to this factor alone accomplishes little."[80]

And in his paper "The relationship of the diet to the development of atherosclerosis in man," Keys made his views unambiguous: "The evidence—both from experiments and from field surveys—indicates that the cholesterol content, per se, of all natural diets has *no* significant effect on either the serum cholesterol level or the development of atherosclerosis in man."

Cholesterol: Killer or Falsely Accused?

At its ten-year follow-up, a strong, statistically significant correlation emerged between the men's average cholesterol levels and their rate of death from heart disease—an *r-value* of 0.80. You may remember from our discussion in *The Hitchhiker's Guide to Nutritional Research* that an *r-value* in statistics is known as the *correlation coefficient*—a measure of the linear relationship between two things, potentially ranging anywhere from -1 (a perfect inverse relationship) to 1 (a perfect positive relationship). Here, an *r-value* of 0.80 is high enough to be noteworthy.

Yet buried in that strong association was a more nuanced picture. In fact, the "it's complicated" theme held true for the study as a whole—and Chapman, the writer who penned the foreword for *Seven Countries*, even outright stated that the study's findings "deflate the evangelical hysteria" of those who think they can live a century or more if only they eliminate all those pesky risk factors for disease.[14]

Part of the problem was that few patterns held true for all of the study's cohorts, casting doubt on the potential of heart disease to be a black-and-white issue with an equally clear-cut solution. And when it came to blood cholesterol, even that statistically strong link with heart disease concealed a much deeper story. For instance, the study's ten-year follow-up unearthed the following nuggets.

- In Croatia, there was "no discernable tendency" for cholesterol level to correlate with any form of heart disease among the study's participants.[15]

- In Italy, the link between higher cholesterol and incidence of heart disease was fairly weak compared to Finland or the Netherlands.[16]

- In Serbia, the relationship between cholesterol levels and heart disease incidence failed to reach statistical significance.[17]

- In the Tanushimaru cohort in Japan, average cholesterol levels rose over 40 mg/dL between 1958 and 1999 (along with blood pressure and body mass index rising in step), but heart disease rates remained low.[18]

- Among American railroad workers, those whose cholesterol levels landed in the top quintile (that is, the highest 20 percent) ended up dying of heart disease at a rate almost four times greater than men in the bottom quintile. But for everybody else, cholesterol levels and heart disease mortality simply weren't related.[19] In other words, *it was only among the highest of the high that cholesterol seemed linked with cardiovascular problems*— casting significant doubt on the idea that "the lower, the better" applies to cholesterol targets.

- Despite its citizens' near immunity from heart disease, the average cholesterol level in Crete was 206.9 mg/dL—a value considered "borderline high" by today's mainstream guidelines.[20]

Ultimately, it seemed total cholesterol bore *some* sort of relationship with heart disease—but the pattern didn't creep up until a fairly high threshold. In contrast to what you might hear at a doctor's office today, Keys summarized the study's findings as showing that "at blood serum levels below 220 mg/dl or so, cholesterol is not a significant factor" for heart disease.[21] The description Keys gave in his 1980 *Seven Countries* publication nails the inconsistency of high blood cholesterol as a risk factor:

A WEIGHTY ISSUE

Along with its scroll of other findings, the Seven Countries Study also slaughtered a few sacred cows—including the role of body weight and obesity in heart disease.

The data collected after the first ten years determined that, at least on a statistical level, neither relative weight nor body fat had much to do with the men's differing rates of heart disease or total mortality. Or as Keys put it: "In none of the areas of this study was overweight or obesity a major risk factor for death or the incidence of coronary heart disease."[81]

In fact, for most of the study's cohorts, the probability of dying "appeared to be *least* for the men somewhat *over* the average in relative weight or fatness" (emphasis mine).[82]

In other words, not only did heart disease seem unrelated to a person's weight, but men who were a bit on the heavier side actually had the best odds of staying alive—at least in the ten-year window after the study first launched.

Of course, the study couldn't rule out the possibility that chronic diseases, such as cancer, had caused the lower body weights, consequently giving the false impression that higher body weight was "protective"—a conundrum we still need more research to solve.

Even today, the body weight-heart disease link continues to stir up controversy. In May of 2013, Harvard researcher Walter Willett landed in hot water after calling one study "a pile of rubbish" because it suggested overweight people had a longevity advantage over their slimmer counterparts.[83] *Nature*, the journal that published the original study, shot back with an editorial saying it's "risky to oversimplify science for the sake of a clear public-health message."[84]

The ten-year experience of the Seven Countries Study indicates that the importance of serum cholesterol as a risk factor varies among populations. In populations with a high frequency of coronary heart disease, the incidence of the disease, especially of death and infarction [heart attack], tends to be directly related to the serum cholesterol level. In populations in which the disease is relatively uncommon, the cholesterol level in the blood seems to have much less, or even no, prognostic significance.[22]

Let's review. We can see that cholesterol only seems to be a risk factor in certain contexts: within populations plagued with heart disease. Elsewhere, folks with higher cholesterol levels don't seem to be at greater risk from the disease. That anomaly suggests several possibilities:

1. That a third variable (or cluster of variables) drives up both heart disease rates and cholesterol concentration.

2. That other factors need to be in place in order to turn cholesterol into something harmful—factors absent in regions where high cholesterol fails to line up with heart disease risk.

3. That other components of diet and lifestyle offset the impact of high cholesterol in some populations, even if it *does* carry an inherent risk when considered in isolation.

Although none of those possibilities are either mutually exclusive or definitive, they all point to the fact that high cholesterol, in and of itself, is only a small part of the heart disease equation. (Indeed, as our understanding of cholesterol has advanced, we now know that total cholesterol—in most cases—reveals less about the state of your body than do markers like HDL, LDL, and triglycerides.)

And if we shine our researcher's light away from heart disease and onto other aspects of health, the Seven Countries Study reveals some even more intriguing discoveries: in a 2002 analysis of the Seven Countries Study's surviving Finnish men, both low total cholesterol and low LDL cholesterol were associated with significantly *greater* levels of depression.[23] That trend stuck around even after adjusting for weight change and chronic disease. As the researchers noted, their study "is the first to show an independent association of low LDL-cholesterol concentration with a high amount of depressive symptoms" in the elderly.

Here are some more juicy tidbits to chew on: In Finland, men with higher cholesterol at the beginning of the study had *lower* risk of dying from everything other than heart disease.[24] As Keys put it in his 1980 *Seven Countries* publication, "the lowest serum cholesterol concentrations at entry were associated with an excessive ten-year death rate from causes other than coronary heart disease."[25] Those with higher cholesterol levels were actually living longer, regardless of heart disease trends.

Want more? Check out what else Keys learned from his study:

- In Italy and Greece, the ten-year death rate from all causes tended to *decrease* with higher cholesterol levels.[26] Again, *the folks with higher cholesterol levels had greater longevity.*

- Among the study as a whole, an inverse relationship ($r= -0.34$) popped up when correlating average cholesterol levels to deaths from causes other than heart disease.[27]

- In the study's Corfu cohort, where cancer was a leading cause of death, serum cholesterol levels between 183 and 218 mg/dL had a "protective" effect on cancer over the course of forty years— meaning folks who started out with cholesterol levels within that range were the least likely to die of cancer during the next four decades.[28] That's right, *lower cholesterol is associated with greater cancer mortality.*

Keys elaborated on this last finding in *Seven Countries,* sliding in a factoid likely to irk statin companies today:

> From the evidence it appears that the serum cholesterol concentration is an important risk factor for the incidence of coronary heart disease at levels of perhaps 220 mg/dl or more. At levels below 200 mg/dl, decreasing cholesterol concentrations tend to be associated with increasing rates of non-coronary death.[29]

Later in the publication, Keys drove home the point about low-cholesterol risks even further. Take special note of the last sentence.

The consideration of the American experience, with the customary assumption of linear relationships, has led to the view that the lower the cholesterol concentration, the better for the individual and the public health, a view endangered by concentration on coronary heart disease and the current situation in the United States. That view would appear to have serious limitations for other populations.[30]

So what does all this mean? Even though the Seven Countries Study made a decent case for high cholesterol levels increasing heart disease risk (at least past a certain threshold), the story changes when we look at other forms of death. We'll see in an upcoming chapter, too, how attempts to coax down cholesterol through diet have done little to improve overall mortality. This highlights the importance of looking at the big picture instead of focusing myopically on a single disease or health outcome.

The Mediterranean Diet

Along with securing saturated fat and blood cholesterol as creatures to be feared, the Seven Countries Study gave birth to the popular "Mediterranean diet" you've probably seen splashed across headlines, book titles, and magazine covers in recent years. In fact, Keys himself had been so inspired by the remarkable health of some of the Mediterranean cohorts that he ended up promoting a diet based on their eating patterns, authoring a book in 1975 called *How to Eat Well and Stay Well the Mediterranean Way*. That said, the "Mediterranean diet" we talk about today is somewhat of a misnomer. Consider the number of countries bordering the Mediterranean—all with diverse traditional cuisines. To be sure, referring to *the* Mediterranean diet is like referring to *the* breed of cat, or *the* Cezanne painting, or *the* Beatles song. There are actually quite a few variations of all the above.

Yet some of the Mediterranean regions also proved to be the most confounding for the study, and may have, over the years, unduly influenced the ideas we've gleaned from its data. Let's move on now and take a look at why.

A Big Fat Greek Oversight

Out of all the cohorts in Keys's study, the sunny Greek island of Crete emerged as the most shining of stars. Its men enjoyed longer life expectancies and lower heart disease rates than any other region under the Seven Countries' watch. And the local diet seemed easy enough to credit for that: a cuisine brimming with wild vegetables, sun-ripened fruits, fresh fish, handpicked nuts and pulses, and the ambrosial nectar we know as olive oil—what's not to love about that?

As it turned out, quite a few things. Just as the critics picked apart Keys's Six Countries Analysis, some had similar qualms with the Seven Countries Study's portrayal of Cretan cuisine. In a 2004 paper, *World Nutrition* editor Geoffrey Cannon pointed out a glaring omission involving that famed Greek island: the impact of local religion on eating habits, especially in the study's most spectacular longevity pockets. "Curiously," Cannon wrote, "and all the more so given his previous epic Minnesota Study on energy restriction, Dr. Keys overlooked a relevant factor: the practice, still common especially in rural mainland Greek and Cretan communities, of fasting."[31]

In Greece, the predominant religion is Orthodox Christianity—a faith with a two-thousand-year-old fasting tradition that involves abstaining from olive oil, all animal products except shellfish and snails, and alcohol for just more than 180 days per year (with some exceptions made depending on the fasting period, especially for fish and dairy).[32,33] That includes following special fasting rules almost every Wednesday and Friday of the week, during the forty days of Lent, and throughout other holy periods encompassing many weeks of the year.

As Cannon noted, the fasting periods also result in about a 10 percent drop in calorie intake—a significant finding, given the speculation surrounding energy restriction and longevity.[34] Existing studies of the Greek Orthodox have also shown that, while fasting, they have a lower intake of trans fats, but a higher intake of fruits, vegetables, legumes, fiber, magnesium, and folate compared to non-fasting control groups.[35,36] Perhaps not surprisingly, their risk factors for heart disease and other conditions plummet accordingly: Orthodox fasters boast lower LDL cholesterol, an improved LDL to HDL ratio, and lower body mass indexes relative to non-fasters.[37]

Although the Orthodox's intermittent abstinence from oils and most animal foods could—from one angle—be used to argue the benefits of lowfat, low-calorie, vegetarian eating, the health perks of their fasting periods could actually be due to quite a few different variables:

- A higher intake of beneficial plant compounds (regardless of reduction in animal food intake)

- Increased consumption of omega-3-rich snails and mineral-dense shellfish

- Cyclical restriction of protein (fasting)

- Replacement of isolated oils with higher-nutrient whole foods

- Moderate alcohol consumption

And plowing even deeper, Cannon raised another possible connection between the Orthodox fasting practices and their sparkling health outcomes:

> I propose that fasting … itself allows the body to rest and recuperate, just as the practice of meditation and reflection during a period of fasting refreshes the spirit. This introduces the provocative possibility that states of mind induced during times of religious observance, of which fasting is traditionally an integral part, are reciprocally beneficial to physical health, and so are nourishing in the broadest sense of the word.[38]

Despite the clear significance of fasting on health and longevity, the Seven Countries Study—both in its Crete cohort and elsewhere—failed to differentiate between participants who followed traditional fasting rituals and those who did not. After reading Cannon's paper, two Cretan researchers contacted Christos Aravins—the man who'd been responsible for carrying out the Seven Countries Study in Greece—and confirmed that in the 1960s, when the study's dietary data were collected, 60 percent of the participants there had been following Orthodox fasting rules and modifying their diets accordingly.[39]

"It is indeed the case that this was not noted in the study, and no attempt was made to differentiate between fasters and non-fasters," wrote the researchers. In their view, the oversight was a remarkable and troublesome omission:

> It still remains unknown whether the results of the Seven Countries Study in Crete, which have been very widely cited and have crucially influenced dietary guidelines and industrial practices all over the world, were about olive oil in particular, the Mediterranean diet in general—or the beneficial effects of fasting.... From our own recent studies, we are sure that the effects on serum lipids and longevity of fasting according to Greek Orthodox Church practices would have been significant, if relative data had been made available in the Seven Countries Study.

More than any other cohort, Crete's ninja-like evasion of heart disease and impressive longevity influenced our current perspectives on diet. Its low intake of saturated fat and fabulous health outcomes also reinforced, by the sheer power of math, a statistical correlation between saturated fat and heart disease in the Seven Countries Study's data.

So how would the study's famous results have changed if Crete's fasting patterns had been taken into account? Without viewing the full picture from Keys's day, we may never know.

A Sweet Smackdown

To supporters of the diet-heart hypothesis, Keys is nothing short of a hero. But more recently, the view of Keys as a somewhat malevolent, anti-science nemesis has been put forth by a number of diet books and other resources challenging mainstream ideas about nutrition. It's mighty tempting to cast historical figures as *good* versus *evil* for the sake of storytelling—but rarely is the past so clear-cut.

And Keys, regardless of the argument that he steered nutrition onto shaky ground, certainly fell into a gray zone. To help strip away the black-and-white portrayal often haunting this man, let's take a look at his long-standing battle with another player of his era: British physiologist John Yudkin, who, like Keys, fills the role of neither hero nor crank.

In fact, the men's professional paths followed an eerily similar trajectory: both had been hot on the heart disease trail since the 1950s, when researchers first noticed its prevalence suddenly surging. Keys and Yudkin both formed their earliest theories by correlating international dietary habits with mortality rates; both ruffled food industry feathers; and both spent their lives trying to convince the world of a heart disease theory they wholly believed was true. And they both wrote books that aired their long-standing grievances with each other.

How could two brilliant minds with so much in common be embroiled in such a bitter, intellectual duel, you ask? The answer lies in their wildly different vantage points. Where Keys saw fat as the villain, Yudkin found another beast entirely: sugar.

Yudkin's first public indictment of sugar and heart disease came in 1957, when—in a move evocative of Keys's 1953 "perfect curve" graph—he plotted the sugar intake of fifteen countries against each nation's rate of heart disease mortality. Just as Keys had seen with fat, Yudkin saw an alarming parallel between sugar consumption and cardiac deaths. And just as Keys had *done* with fat, Yudkin promptly started prodding correlation for signs of causation.

And his efforts weren't without some success.

Although nutritionists at the time made little distinction between starch and sugar in the diet—operating under the assumption that it all turned into glucose in the bloodstream—Yudkin published some of the earliest research exploring their different metabolic effects.[40]

In 1964, he coauthored a *Lancet* paper showing that patients with severely plaque-filled arteries tend to eat about twice as much sugar as folks with healthier hearts.[41] (Although critics like Keys pointed out that not all heart disease patients had a high sugar intake, Yudkin retorted—emphasis his—that "*no one* has ever shown any difference in *fat* consumption between people with and without coronary disease, but this has in no way deterred Dr. Keys and his followers."[42])

And at a time when the blood marker du jour was cholesterol, Yudkin turned his focus to insulin, blood glucose, and triglycerides.[43] His research eventually made his suspicions about sugar sprout into a full-blown conviction that the sweet, white granules were at least partially driving the heart disease epidemic. And in contrast to the cholesterol-centrism of Keys's theory, Yudkin believed the root of cardiovascular disease lay in hormonal disturbances in the body—most notably with the way the pancreas produces insulin.[44]

Drawing from observational data, animal experiments, human trials, and biochemistry much in the same way Keys had done, Yudkin found the evidence compelling enough to warn: "If only a small fraction of what is already known about the effects of sugar were to be revealed in relation to any other material used as a food additive, the material would promptly be banned."

Along with synthesizing modern-day evidence, Yudkin also crafted his theory in the light of evolutionary logic. "It *does* matter that your diet is now very likely to be different from that which has been evolved over millions of years as the diet most suitable for you as a member of the species *Homo sapiens,*" he wrote in his well-received book *Pure, White and Deadly*—published in 1972, with updated editions in 1986 and 2012.[45]

Operating off his era's now largely outdated anthropological evidence, Yudkin describes the diet of early humans as a thing of much meat, with minimal sweetness.

> In order to survive, *africanus* [an early hominid] had to forsake the vegetarian and fruitarian existence … and change to a scavenging and hunting existence that was largely carnivorous. … In nutritional terms, the diet of prehistoric human beings and their ancestors during perhaps two million years or more was rich in protein, moderately rich in fat, and usually poor in carbohydrate.[46]

Today, we know the dietary patterns of the past two million years involved something far more nuanced than chest-thumping cavemen dragging mastodon thighs back to their lairs. Rather than a universal main course, meat intake may have varied tremendously depending on geography, season, climate, and other environmental influences; and diets were unlikely to be "poor" in carbohydrate once the control of fire made roots and tubers more edible.[47]

At the time of Yudkin's writing, however, the "historical carnivore" image helped sculpt his views about where the modern diet had gone wrong—leading him to the stance that sugar, a relative scarcity during evolution, was a much more likely culprit in modern disease than was fat or animal products, which had been consumed for millions of years without apparent harm. In sum, Yudkin built his theory on five pieces of evidence:

- The unprecedented intake of sugar clashing with anything the human body had experienced before the Neolithic era

- The strong correlation between sugar consumption and heart disease deaths in various countries

- The increase in sugar intake over the years paralleling the increase in cardiac mortality

- The observation that men with heart disease tend to be hefty consumers of sugar

- And the possibility that sugar raises triglycerides, insulin levels, blood glucose, and even serum cholesterol

The collection of arguments bore such close resemblance to those Keys used for saturated fat that Yudkin, naturally, thought his American counterpart had overlooked a critical possibility: that heart disease was killing people sweetly rather than greasily. Of those promoting the saturated fat theory of heart disease (and letting sugar off the hook), Yudkin called Keys "the most important and certainly the most dogmatic research worker."[48]

Like two cars playing chicken, Keys's fat-centric theory and Yudkin's sugar-centric one raced boldly toward a one-lane bridge of scientific consensus—both determined to reach that narrow road before his rival. Although neither theory was as strong as either man wished, Yudkin's, figuratively speaking, was the first to swerve, driven off path by inconsistent data and a mob of contemporaries already sold on the danger of saturated fat. Despite enjoying some popularity in the 1960s and 1970s, his theory had spun its wheels in the gutter by the time the USDA Food Guide Pyramid immortalized fat as the true dietary demon.

The idea that sugar could be a problem for anything other than tooth decay wouldn't return to mainstream thought for decades. As Yudkin relayed in his book *Pure, White and Deadly,* a sugar industry advertisement captured the era's sentiment well—that sugar was actually a *boon* for weight loss and appetite control. Here's a sampling of the bold claims found in those advertisements:

"Willpower fans, the search is over!"

"And guess where it's at? In sugar!"

"Sugar works faster than any other food to turn
your appetite down, turn energy up."

"Spoil your appetite with sugar,
and you could come up with willpower."

"Sugar—only 18 calories per teaspoon, and it's all energy."[49]

A paper from the 1970 *Bulletin of the World Health Organization*,
penned by Dr. Roberto Masironi, had also scored a point in favor of
Keys (and consequently, away from Yudkin). Masironi had plotted
heart disease mortality data for thirty-seven countries against each
nation's intake of total fat, saturated fat, sucrose, total simple sugars,
complex carbohydrates, and protein.[50]

Of that flavorful variable soup, only fat and saturated fat emerged
as having high, positive correlations with heart disease rates. Sugar's
correlation, on the other hand, was fairly weak. Masironi concluded
that the results were "in line with the generally accepted hypothesis
that excessive intake of fats, especially the saturated type, may have a
detrimental effect on cardiovascular health."

So what went wrong? Why were Masironi's findings different?

Masironi explained it as just a matter of country choice. In those
earlier sugar-incriminating studies, the data had been pulled mostly
from Europe, where sugar intake didn't vary much among the various
countries. The range was from about 13 percent of total calories for
the lowest-consuming nation to 21 percent for the highest. Do the
math: that's a range of only 8 percent. The noteworthy association
seen there didn't hold up when more geographical variety was added
to the mix. Here's Masironi:

> … in the 37 countries considered in the present investigation sim-
> ple sugar consumption ranges from 5.1% to 38.5% of the total
> calorie intake. As there are countries, such as Colombia, Costa Rica,
> Jordan, Mexico and others, where death rates from atherosclerotic

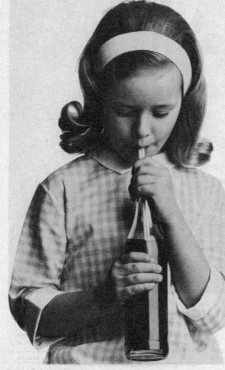

Fig. 9. One of many ads dispensed by the sugar industry to encourage Americans—including children—to eat more refined sugar.

heart disease (AHD) are low and yet the calorie contribution from simple sugars is as high as, or even higher than in the European countries, then we may assume that the relation between AHD death rates and simple sugar intake … is actually a secondary association for which a causal significance has not been proved yet.[51]

In other words, shoveling more countries into the statistical furnace only smothered the association seen within Europe. Sugar was probably just riding the tail of something more directly involved in heart disease, Masironi suggested.

Now, remember our earlier discussion on Yerushalmy and Hilleboe and the data they found that correlates increasing wealth with heart disease? Keep that in mind as you read on.

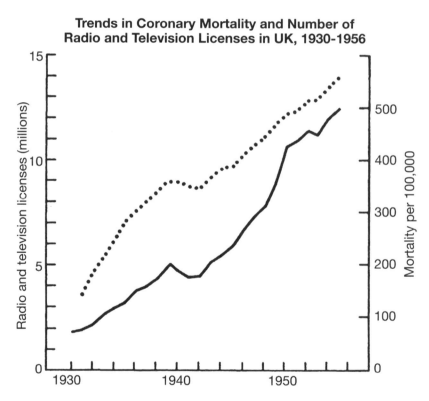

Trends in Coronary Mortality and Number of Radio and Television Licenses in UK, 1930-1956

TABLE 5. Broken line represents number of deaths from heart attack per 100,000 people; solid line represents number of radios and televisions owned in the UK. (Source: *Pure, White and Deadly*, John Yudkin, 1972.)

Masironi's data also showed heart disease climbing hand in hand with national per capita income and calorie intake. The pattern reinforced two things: the idea that *elements of affluence may form a toxic cocktail for heart disease*. And: that *saturated fat could be an indication of affluence rather than a cause of the diseases it accompanies*. Masironi raised the possibility in his own words, explaining:

> Higher consumption of fats (particularly of the saturated type) and of refined sugars, and lower consumption of complex carbohydrates are usually associated with higher prosperity. ... Therefore, it may well be that the relation between dietary factors and incidence of AHD [atherosclerotic heart disease] is secondary to other factors, which are in turn associated with living standards, and which perhaps play a more important role.

Masironi went on to suggest that there could be a sort of symbiosis between diet and lifestyle, and that a certain "way of life may cause the dietary factors to be harmful for some populations while they are harmless for others." We'll revisit that idea in a short while, so sit tight.

The "it's not really saturated fat *or* sugar" notion gained additional support when Masironi conducted a deeper analysis of the thirty-seven countries' data—this time exploring whether the rise in cardiovascular mortality over the years was paralleling any dietary shifts happening at the same time. Correlating each nation's death ratio between 1955 and 1965 with changes in food intake over a similar period, the time-based analysis showed the factor most strongly linked with increasing rates of heart disease was the rise in total calorie availability ($r = 0.57$)—perhaps the strongest dietary marker for national affluence. Saturated fat intake, on the other hand, was slightly *negatively* associated with those escalating cardiac deaths ($r = -0.27$), whereas sucrose and simple sugar intake were positively correlated, but to a lesser degree than calories in general ($r = 0.42$ and $r = 0.40$, respectively). The picture painted was a clear one: *access to greater levels of food seemed more pertinent on the heart-disease front than did any particular diet constituent*—whether as a causative agent or yet another reflection of national affluence.

Yudkin himself had also stumbled across the tight linkage between affluence and heart disease. In fact, he noted something significant in the multi-country graphs that he and Keys had both produced in the 1950s. On one hand, he spotted a "moderate but by no means excellent" relationship between fat consumption and coronary mortality, and a slightly stronger relationship with sugar. But the most robust relationship of all, he found, was between the rise in the number of reported coronary deaths and the rise in ownership of radio and television sets.[52] That last point might seem like a classic example of *correlation doesn't equal causation*—after all, how could a noise-producing box clog your arteries? Yet Yudkin implored readers to keep an open mind:

> The factors that have been implicated in causing coronary thrombosis include several that are associated with affluence—sedentariness, obesity, cigarette smoking, fat consumption, sugar consumption. On the one hand, therefore, the incidence of coronary thrombosis will be higher in those countries in which there is greater affluence as measured by any index such as cigarette or fat consumption, but also by the number of television sets or motorcars or telephones. On the other hand, many of these indices of affluence are likewise indices of sedentariness.[53]

Yudkin's observation is the same one that led us to label our "new" wave of chronic conditions—from heart disease to certain cancers to diabetes to obesity—as "diseases of affluence." Regardless of their specific cause, they seem to tag along with national wealth and the luxuries, both edible and lifestyle related, that accompany it. Among those tangled affluence-related variables, Yudkin had seen sugar as the problem; Keys had seen saturated fat; and other researchers had seen everything from smoking to sedentariness to overconsumption of food in general.

Nonetheless, Masironi *did* throw a bone to Yudkin's sugar theory despite lack of support within his thirty-seven-country analysis. Along with consistent links popping up between heart disease, diabetes, and sugar intolerance, Masironi noted:

SUGAR BULLIES

No big surprise here: the sugar industry launched a media attack against John Yudkin's book *Pure, White and Deadly*. In 1979, the *Quarterly Bulletin of the World Sugar Research Organization* (WRSO) published "For your dustbin," which read:

> Pure, White and Deadly. J. Yudkin. Davis-Poynter Ltd, London 1972. Readers of science fiction will no doubt be distressed to learn that according to the publishers the above work is out of print and no longer obtainable.[91]

The "science fiction" jab spurred Yudkin to take legal action for libel, launching a four-year exchange with lawyers until the sugar organization finally agreed to publish a retraction and pay his legal costs.[92]

As regards the relationship of sugars to cardiovascular diseases it must be borne in mind that these nutrients have common metabolic pathways with fats. Disturbances in carbohydrate metabolism may be responsible for abnormal fat metabolism and may therefore act as a causative factor in the development of atherosclerosis and of coronary disease.

(It remained unknown, however, whether sugar itself was responsible for disrupting carbohydrate metabolism on its own, or whether it simply exacerbated the problem once those disturbances were already in place.)

Whether casting saturated fat or sugar or any other food component as a suspect, though, Masironi's data couldn't prove anything definitive about those nutrients' roles in heart disease—in the same way causality is hands-off territory for *any* observational data.

As should be abundantly clear by now, the *correlation doesn't equal causation* dictum is a particularly important one to keep in mind when studying uncontrolled data at the population level. And what's more, like both Keys and Yudkin had done previously, Masironi drew his data from FAO food balance sheets—which show how much food is *available* for human consumption in each country, instead of how much is actually consumed. The latter requires a fair bit of guesswork and theoretical number crunching, rather than the more telling methods of following folks around and monitoring every morsel they put into their mouths. (Masironi conceded the sheets were a "crude estimate" of food consumption, but felt they yielded data close enough to that produced by more controlled analyses to be trustworthy.)

What's more, Masironi noted that the increase in heart disease itself was—at least in part—"likely to be an artifact brought about by the changing fashion in certifying heart disease as a cause of death," thanks to better diagnostic procedures. Given that medical care tends to improve as a nation's affluence increases, it's quite possible the wealth-and-heart-disease connection gained a boost from doctors merely getting better at finding it.

But none of those issues—from national affluence to diagnostic changes to non-dietary lifestyle components—deterred either Keys or Yudkin from their respective theories. And with Keys's take on heart disease developing its own gravitational force of support (even when the data didn't necessarily warrant it), Yudkin's voice eventually faded into background noise. Keys remained stalwart in his belief that saturated fat was the true culprit in heart disease, and that sugar—despite Yudkin's protests to the contrary—was an innocent bystander.

Thus began the dramatic professional duel between Yudkin and Keys. In 1971, Keys published a paper in the journal *Atherosclerosis* titled "Sucrose in the diet and coronary heart disease," declaring point-blank that the sugar-heart disease theory "is not supported by acceptable clinical, epidemiological, theoretical or experimental evidence."[54] The paper, essentially a polemic against Yudkin, was largely a case of the pot calling the kettle black. Keys chastised Yudkin for precisely the same maneuvers he'd used to build the empire of evidence he raised against saturated fat, writing that Yudkin: (1) selectively chose countries to support his hypothesis when a much larger pool of data was available; (2) used unreliable food disappearance figures; and (3) prematurely declared that heart disease was "more closely associated with the level of sugar consumption than with the level of any other dietary component."

However, Keys did whip out something Yudkin couldn't defeat at the time: a freshly plucked bouquet of evidence from the Seven Countries Study. Keys argued that the results of the international, prospective cohort study he'd spearheaded were far more meaningful than Yudkin's comparison of diet and mortality statistics—and its latest analysis seemed to confirm that saturated fat trounced sugar as a heart threat. Although Keys conceded that sugar and heart disease *were* correlated in the data, with an *r-value* of 0.78 for percent of calories from sugar and heart disease deaths, he insisted it was only because sugar tagged closely alongside saturated fat intake (a correlation of $r= 0.84$ between the two) and thus looked guilty by association. Keys believed the tendency for saturated fat and sugar to accompany each other in people's diets was "adequate to explain the observed relationship between sucrose and CHD" without having to resort to the idea that sugar actually played a role in the disease.

But the deepest cut to Yudkin's theory was a slightly more sophisticated analysis of the Seven Countries data. Keys explained that when the influence of saturated fat was mathematically muted—an effort to remove it as a confounder and see the role of other diet variables more clearly—the sugar-heart disease link dwindled to insignificance; but when using the same method to adjust for sugar intake, the saturated fat-heart disease link persisted. In his *Atherosclerosis* paper, Keys referenced a finding he also wrote about in *Seven Countries: A Multivariate Analysis of Death and Coronary Disease:*

> Partial correlation analysis showed that, with dietary saturated fat held constant, the correlation between dietary sucrose and the incidence of coronary heart disease is not significant ($r= 0.13$). On the other hand, with sucrose held constant in the partial correlation analysis, the correlation of the coronary incidence rate with the mean percentage of calories from saturated fat is 0.62.[55]

In other words, it appeared saturated fat was indeed running the show, mathematically speaking—creating a false correlation between sugar and heart disease simply because of the way the study's diet variables were tangled. As Keys gladly pointed out, it also didn't help Yudkin's case that other researchers had failed to replicate his findings that coronary patients were eating substantially more sugar than their healthy counterparts, particularly in larger, better-designed studies.[56] In all, Keys felt Yudkin had "no theoretical basis or experimental evidence" to support his sugar theory. "But the propaganda keeps on reverberating," Keys wrote, ultimately concluding:

None of what is said here should be taken to mean approval of the common high level of sucrose in any diets. But there are plenty of good arguments to reduce the flood of dietary sucrose without building a mountain of nonsense about coronary heart disease.

Incidentally, in 2008, researcher William B. Grant revisited the dietary supply data and heart disease statistics from earlier decades, but—unlike either Keys or Yudkin—included women in his analysis. As he described, his findings showed that animal fat had the highest correlation with heart attacks for males of all age ranges, whereas added sugar had the highest correlation for *females* of all ages.

Grant noted, "Had women been included in the Seven Countries Study, Yudkin might have been able to make a better case for the role of sugar as a risk factor in CHD."[57] Unfortunately, the finding came too late to add fodder to the Keys-Yudkin war in its heyday.

For Keys's part, his 1975 book *How to Eat Well and Stay Well: The Mediterranean Way*—a work inspired by the results of the Seven Countries Study and his long-standing infatuation with Italian health— made sure to drag Yudkin into the conversation for some in-print walloping. Conceding that it'd probably be wise to limit sugar intake due to its paltry nutritional contribution, tendency to promote tooth decay, and hazardousness for diabetics, Keys quickly brought up Yudkin's "unfounded charge" about sugar causing heart disease.

> That charge has been joyfully broadcast all over the world by some elements in the dairy and meat industry; the obvious hope is to divert attention from the effects of dairy and meat fats on the blood cholesterol level, the development of arterial disease, and the clinical consequences of heart attacks on sudden death. ... Among medical scientists Yudkin is alone in his contentions, and the errors in his "evidence" are well documented. ... But Yudkin and his commercial backers are not deterred by the facts; they continue to sing the same discredited tune so a brief answer is needed here.[58]

Continuing, Keys maintained that Yudkin's research with heart disease patients and their sugar intake "would never pass as an acceptable term paper in an undergraduate course in home economics," and that his claim that sugar intake and heart disease rates were closely linked was "utter nonsense."[59] And again returning to accusations once leveled against Keys himself, he complained that "Yudkin selected his countries to support his thesis" and "conveniently omitted [countries] where the diets are highest in sugar but the incidence of heart attacks is notably low."[60] "There is no reason at all to propose that a diet low in sugar will reduce the frequency of heart attacks," Keys concluded.[61]

Incited by the vicious challenges to his theory (and rather embittered personal rivalry), Yudkin shot back with some equally painful swipes at Keys as the years rolled on. Summarizing the existing experiments testing Keys's theory of heart disease, Yudkin noted that most trials swapping out saturated fat for "heart healthy" vegetable oils were hardly worth bragging about. Most failed to improve overall mortality rates, some showed an *increase* in heart disease deaths, and nearly all increased risk of death from certain non-cardiac causes.

The trials that did have promising outcomes were either too poorly designed or too confounder-ridden to be meaningful. "We must conclude," Yudkin wrote, "that all this effort since the 1960s has not succeeded in demonstrating the efficacy of a change in dietary fat in reducing the prevalence of coronary disease."[62] In a 1992 letter in *The Royal Society of Medicine,* Yudkin summed up the failure of those studies to prove Keys's diet-heart hypothesis in even more provocative terms, writing that "Another way of stating these findings is to say that, if you wish to increase the number of people dying from accidents, violence, cancer or strokes, then give them a diet low in cholesterol and fat."[63] (In the next chapter, we'll look at these very studies and see how his assessment wasn't far off the mark.)

Turning to evolution for answers, Yudkin continued to explain—in more theoretical terms—why it wouldn't make sense for industrially processed vegetable oils to be a boon for heart health, per Keys's theory:

> I believe that the best diet for the human species is one made up as far as possible of the foods that were available in our hunting and food-gathering days. The oils rich in polyunsaturates have been available only because of recent advances in agriculture and in the even more recent elaborate industrial techniques of extracting and refining oils; the complex chemical processing of these and other

oils to produce margarine removes this product even further from the sorts of foods available to humanity during millions of years of evolution.[64]

To Yudkin's credit, he remained admirably cautious about confusing his personal views with unflappable proof. In *Pure, White and Deadly,* he warned readers, "Please don't take these statements to imply that I have discovered the secrets of the ideal diet. … I do not mean to imply … that everything I shall be telling you is an absolute certainty."[65]

The epidemiological evidence, he admitted, could not by itself *prove* that sugar—or any other factor—was a cause of heart disease. Rather, it could only offer clues. It was a humility sometimes lacking in his rival Keys's career as he promoted the saturated-fat theory of heart disease with overeager confidence.

Like Keys, Yudkin has been the victim of some history-revising folklore—particularly by those who champion his theory as the correct one, a diamond of truth tragically swept out of sight by Keys's greater clout. In reality, Yudkin was no more a scientific saint than Keys was a heartless villain. While he may have been well ahead of his time in indicting sugar as a problem in the modern diet, its link with heart disease remains indirect at best, and tenuous at worst. Yudkin's data was objectively no stronger than Keys's—and many of the same criticisms delivered by Yerushalmy and Hilleboe applied equally to him. Sugar consumption, as with the consumption of saturated fat and animal products, was a strong surrogate for a country's wealth and modernization; whether it was responsible for damaging hearts or just guilty by association was impossible to tell from observation alone (or from Yudkin's tiny, hard-to-replicate studies of heart disease patients).

What's more, Yudkin *couldn't* discern whether sugar directly caused heart disease or if it merely fanned the flames once the disease's fire was already lit. His first experiments—using only nineteen young men, a fairly small sample size—found that only about a quarter or a third showed "sensitivity" to sugar, as marked by higher insulin levels while consuming a high-sugar diet. "This suggested to us the idea that only a proportion of men are susceptible to coronary thrombosis through eating sugar," Yudkin explained in *Pure, White and Deadly*.[66]

Another of Yudkin's experiments used twenty-seven men, some of whom were patients with vascular disease and the rest of whom were just regular folks coming into a clinic for a checkup.[67] Only among patients who'd already developed the disease did the fasting insulin level correspond with sugar intake; among the healthy clinic visitors, there was no relationship between sugar consumption and insulin. Collectively, the evidence raised the possibility that other factors have to be in place—like metabolic damage from various hazards of the modern lifestyle—in order for sugar to wreak measurable havoc. (As we'll soon see, that may also be the case for saturated fat.)

Further popping the bubble of Yudkin's "suppressed hero" reputation in some circles, modern health enthusiasts might take issue with some claims of his that are often omitted from discussions in his favor. For instance, he wrote that "it really does not matter to your health whether your chicken is produced by the broiler system, or whether you eat potatoes grown with chemical fertilizers"—statements that might ruffle the feathers of those supporting free-range meat and organic farming. And while Yudkin readily derided sugar, he was far more forgiving toward refined starches, claiming in 1978 that there was "little evidence that supports the suggestion that if we ate whole meal bread rather than white bread, we would reduce our chances of developing obesity, coronary heart disease or diabetes."[68]

In all, Yudkin's theory provides important clues about heart disease, introducing new ideas about the role of hormone dysfunction and blood markers other than cholesterol—while also showing there may be more to the industrialized world's disease-promoting diet shifts than saturated fat intake. Yet from an objective standpoint, his theory suffers from many of the same holes found in that of Keys. In the end, both men contributed valuable—but incomplete—ideas into the still-evolving world of heart disease research.

If Not Saturated Fat or Sugar, Then What?

Here's the problem with the theories of both Yudkin and Keys: they each tried to incriminate a single macronutrient without considering the bigger picture. This type of tunnel vision still infects the research world today. Indeed, the context in which saturated fat and sugar are consumed can determine their ultimate effects on one's health. For example, saturated fat may be benign in diets free from industrially processed foods. More and more, the evidence seems to suggest that. But add it to a diet that is swimming in refined grains, excess calories, and high fructose corn syrup, and it might act out of character in health-harming ways. Similarly, it's possible that sugar unleashes its most vicious damage in the context of our modern, highly processed diet.

From that perspective, specific components of diet may not spark disease on their own, but they could potentially fuel it once it's blazing—which means singling out a handful of foods or nutrients, ala current federal recommendations and the researchers that helped usher them into being, might not be enough to halt our most insidious diseases. And if the history of our dietary guidelines is any indication, that certainly seems to be the case. More robust evidence exists for the "food depends on context" argument, and the data continues to mount in this direction.

A 2011 review in *The Netherlands Journal of Medicine* evaluated our collective body of research on saturated fat, carbohydrate, and cardiovascular disease, proposing an intriguing hypothesis about the behavior of saturated fat under different dietary circumstances. Though more research is needed to test it, the theory may reconcile the inconsistencies popping up between clinical studies and epidemiology. The review found that the modern diet tends to promote chronic, low-grade inflammation—a response triggered by damage to your body's tissues. The inflammation then cripples the body's ability to protect itself from other damage. Basically, that chronic inflammation sets the stage for disease.

The paper's authors suggest that dietary saturated fat—while not a health-harming entity in and of itself—may become problematic if it's dumped on top of a soup of inflammation and excess carbohydrate. Such a situation can lead to a buildup of saturated fatty acids in the body, notably as higher levels of free fatty acids in plasma lipids. (Those excess free fatty acids have long been linked with conditions like insulin resistance and diabetes, largely contributing to saturated fat's blacklisted status in the nutrition world.) Explaining the phenomenon, the authors wrote:

> The adverse effects of high SAFA [saturated fatty acid] intake on lipid metabolism are particularly noted when SAFA are combined with a high CHO [carbohydrate] intake. Under these conditions, dietary SAFA are preserved, while the surplus of the consumed CHO is converted to SAFA by hepatic *de novo* fatty acid synthesis.

… Taken together, SAFA accumulate: 1) under eucaloric conditions in normal weight subjects who consume a CHO-rich diet with high glycaemic index; and 2) under hypocaloric conditions in subjects with the metabolic syndrome and non-alcoholic fatty liver disease who consume CHO-rich diets. Thus CHO, particularly those with a high glycaemic index, and pre-existing insulin resistance are confounding factors in the discussion on the relation between CVD [cardiovascular disease] and dietary SAFA.[69]

Don't worry if that explanation is a little dizzying—it's actually fairly simple once we translate the Science-ese. Essentially, eating excess calories in the form of carbohydrates—especially refined carbs, which tend to spike blood sugar levels—kicks off a process called *de novo* fatty acid synthesis: *de novo* ("from the beginning") and fatty acid synthesis (also called "lipogenesis"). That's the enzymatic pathway your body uses to convert dietary carbohydrate into fat.

When you exceed your body's energy needs with a surplus of carbohydrate, it triggers *de novo* lipogenesis. It can also take place even if you don't exceed your energy needs, if the diet is high glycemic and high in carbohydrates. This becomes especially problematic when the scale is tipped in favor of sugar over starch, causing what we call metabolic syndrome, which—encompasses insulin resistance, high triglycerides, high LDL and low HDL cholesterol, and high fasting blood sugar.

This is important stuff! And it bears repeating: ***de novo* lipogenesis can happen even on low-calorie diets that include an excess of high-glycemic carbohydrates.** That means folks with preexisting metabolic problems likely suffer the most from our nationwide low-fat, high-carbohydrate diet advice.

Metabolic syndrome may explain why Yudkin saw "sugar sensitivity" only in a fraction of his patients. That fraction likely already suffered from the condition and had an increased tendency to convert sugar into saturated fat, which then contributed to the blood lipid abnormalities associated with heart disease. More important, though, is the runoff from a high intake of the wrong kinds of carbohydrate—which potentially sets dietary saturated fat on a path for trouble.

Let me explain. Per the review's hypothesis, when you consume a typical Western diet, your body is in a chronic state of inflammation—swimming in the surplus of saturated fatty acids it created from all those excess carbohydrates. Dump a few sticks of butter into the mix and saturated fat may, indeed, worsen the situation. But under such circumstances, blaming saturated fat for heart disease is a bit like blaming a bag of ice for melting everywhere when your freezer door is left open. Given the wrong environment, the behavior that saturated fat takes on could indeed turn damaging—but that's not the fault of saturated fat per se. By ignoring context, we reach some pretty wacky conclusions about the state of affairs and end up blaming the wrong factors.

This could also explain why saturated fat seems to be innocuous in populations with a low-to-naught intake of refined carbohydrates, why high-carbohydrate diets can yield positive health outcomes when fat intake is kept extremely low (such as with the heart-disease-battling programs of doctors Dean Ornish and Caldwell Esselstyn, which we'll examine more closely in chapter eleven, *Herbivore's Dilemma*), why low carbohydrate diets can exert positive effects on cardiovascular indices, and why the standard Western diet—rich in both fat *and* sugar—seems to magnetically attract chronic disease wherever it invades. The interplay of refined carbohydrate and saturated fat creates a brand new beast, one distinctly damaging to the human body.

Simply put, fat and sugar do not make good bedfellows. In fact, our Dutch researchers summed up their findings by calling for a context-dependent revision of our beliefs about saturated fat—especially given its critical interaction with dietary carbohydrate:

> The total body of evidence suggests that attention should be shifted from the harmful effects of dietary SAFA [saturated fatty acids] *per se*, to the prevention of the accumulation of SAFA in body lipids. This shift would emphasize the importance of reducing dietary CHO, especially CHO with a high glycaemic index, rather than reducing dietary SAFA. … Dietary SAFA belong to the many false triggers of inflammation that result from the conflict between our slowly adapting genome and our rapidly changing lifestyle.

Their conclusions sound like a stellar prescription for healthy living: the researchers stated that "more realistic approaches" to fight heart disease include:

- An increase in fish, vegetable, and fruit consumption
- An increase in activity and sleep
- A reduction of high-glycemic carbohydrates, trans fatty acids, and the omega-6 fat linoleic acid
- A reduction in chronic stress

On top of that, genetic factors may play a tremendous role in how each of us responds to saturated fat on an individual level. And chief among those is the ApoE gene.

ApoE4: A Missing Link

Maybe you had a parent, grandparent, or great-grandparent who—after surviving the economic meltdown of the 1930s—developed the remarkable ability to never throw away anything, ever. Stamps, bolts, pennies, tiny watch parts, the snipped-out soles of otherwise desecrated shoes all found a home on a shelf, in a drawer, in a closet, or strewn about the front lawn beside a legion of plastic gnomes. It seems we all know somebody fitting that bill.

If you never experienced times of great shortage, such behavior may have seemed neurotic. But if you'd grown up in the throes of scarcity like your pack-ratting relative did, where squeezing even a dollop of worth out of apparent trash could be a matter of life or death, you, too, might be reluctant to throw out that fifteen-year-old coupon for corn grits.

It just so happens that some of us carry the genetic equivalent of the perpetual hoarder, whose habits stem from much the same reason. Coding a class of apolipoproteins involved in lipid metabolism and dietary cholesterol absorption is the ApoE gene. (Not to be confused with the POE gene, which codes macabre nineteenth-century poetry.)

Depending on what you inherit from your parents, you'll express a combination of any two of the common alleles (or *variants)* for this gene: ApoE2, ApoE3, and ApoE4. It's that last one, ApoE4, that has some peculiar properties when it comes to saturated fat and the hoarding mentality.

Dubbed the "ancestral" allele, it preceded all the others in our evolutionary timeline—a fact that might evoke imagery of meat-eating cavemen who, if anything, would be fantastically equipped to handle a high intake of meat and saturated fat.[70] Actually, the ApoE4 allele is even *older*. Studies of nonhuman primates like chimpanzees, bonobos, and red vervet monkeys show they all carry the form of ApoE that resembles ApoE4 in humans, and unlike us, don't have any alternative versions of the gene popping up within each species.[71, 72, 73] That suggests that ApoE4 (or something convincingly close to it) dates *way* back to our early primate ancestors, existing before the human-chimpanzee split that happened at least five million years ago. In fact, it likely wasn't until the last two hundred thousand years or so—squarely in the middle Paleolithic—that the other ApoE alleles first spread en masse.[74]

So what does that mean for ApoE4 carriers? Its modus operandi—sculpted by so many years of evolution—is to save, squeeze, and stockpile. ApoE4 never got the memo that many of us are living in dietary abundance now, and it has no "off" switch to quell its hoarding ways.

Chiseled by the challenging conditions it emerged from, ApoE4 excels at squeezing every last drop of benefit from nutrient-dense foods—which, back in the times of our very early ancestors, were in short or inconsistent supply. Even in more recent hunter-gatherer groups, where ApoE4 also tends to appear with unusual frequency, food often comes in feast and famine cycles—making it imperative to glean as much nutrition from meat and other dense fare when those foods are in abundance.

Historically, ApoE4 would have been a boon in parts of the globe (and eras of history) where certain pathogens are abundant. A number of parasites, fungi, and other microscopic organisms can actually slurp up lipoproteins from human blood—a sort of gang-like stripping of car parts—to use for themselves. The result can be ultra-low cholesterol levels for the human host, making ApoE4, with its cholesterol-hoarding tendencies, something of a godsend.

All that said, it's in situations of shortage, unpredictability, and high infection and parasite load that ApoE4 shines brightest: it helps prevent cholesterol levels from dipping *too* low in times of nutritional scarcity, and boosts survival by maximizing the body's ability to suction up fat and cholesterol from the diet.

But in a modern context, ApoE4 is more of a burden than a boon. Due to its unique effect on lipid metabolism, folks carrying at least one copy of ApoE4 have significantly higher rates of heart disease and Alzheimer's (a condition fascinatingly linked with cholesterol) than folks with no E4 alleles, as well as notably higher LDL levels.[75,76] ApoE4 carriers also appear to be more prone to inflammation and oxidative stress than the rest of the population.[77] And worse, some human studies—albeit observational—support the idea that a high saturated fat intake might increase heart attack risk for ApoE4 carriers, especially for folks stuck with two copies of the allele.[78]

Even if you carry the ApoE4 gene, it doesn't mean dietary cholesterol and fat are cruel substances out to kill you. Quite the contrary: your body views them as such precious resources that it strives to soak up as much of them from your diet as possible—just as a dehydrated desert wanderer might try to salvage a few rare drops of water from a barrel cactus.

But due to that unstoppable "nutritional hoarding," it may well be that ApoE4 carriers do best on diets that emphasize leaner animal products—a nutrition profile resembling the protein-rich insects, small mammals, reptiles, and scavenged fare encountered by our distant hominoid ancestors, in the days before food supply was more constant. Likewise, intermittent consumption of saturated-fat, cholesterol-rich food, in the sporadic way many hunter-gatherer groups consume it, may offer some perks for ApoE4 carriers, in contrast to a steady and consistent intake of such foods.

And even when such diets boast success for many adherents, ApoE4 carriers may find they respond poorly to eating plans like the Atkins diet, Paleolithic-style diets emphasizing fatty meat and coconut oil, or other cuisines with ample fat and cholesterol content.

The genotype-specific responses to saturated fat intake may, indeed, help explain the inconsistencies we see in observational studies about saturated fat intake and blood cholesterol. Unfortunately, very few studies looking at diet and heart disease—and virtually none of the most famous and influential ones—documented participants' ApoE type. To boot, this is just one of a number of genetic variations that influence fat and cholesterol metabolism.

Modern Living and an Old Indian Proverb

Perhaps the greatest casualty of the diet-heart hypothesis, as perpetuated through the figures and studies we've explored in this chapter, was its destruction of a once-holistic perspective of food. Post Keys, we no longer saw our sustenance as a symbiosis of nutrients

—but instead started defining items on the basis of a single macronutrient they contained, particularly fat or saturated fat. The Keysian mindset led, directly or indirectly, to our current reductionist view of eating, where trigger terms like *saturated fat* or *cholesterol* or *fiber* or *omega-3* or *antioxidants* tell us immediately (and often erroneously) whether a food is good or bad for us. And with that mentality came a prime opportunity to exploit our newly warped, simplistic view of our very sustenance for the purposes of marketing, profit, fear, and manipulation.

But perhaps Keys and Yudkin had both been right in their own way. The combination of highly refined carbohydrates like sugar, energy excess bestowed by increased food availability, and a higher intake of saturated-fat-rich foods—combined with high-stress inflammatory lifestyles of the modern world—create the perfect storm for heart disease. (Of course, the true contribution of either saturated fat or sugar to that mess remains impossible to untangle from observational data.)

Genetic variation, virtually absent from either Keys's or Yudkin's research, may likewise have explained the anomalies and inconsistencies both of their theories generated on a global scale.

In reviewing the research, an old proverb from India comes to mind. It tells the story of a group of blind men trying to understand an elephant—each groping around a different part of its large and diversely angled body, struggling to perceive what exactly the animal is.

A man feeling the elephant's leg thinks the creature resembles a tree; a man feeling its ears believes it's like a fan; a man feeling its tail declares the elephant to dangle like a rope. The truth about the elephant, of course, is that it's all of those things and then some—a compilation of sundry parts, united to form an entity greater than a single limb or trunk alone. All the blind men in the tale are right as well as wrong.

So it goes with Keys and Yudkin. They'd each stumbled upon a piece of the puzzle, but failed to see a broader landscape of which it was a part. Higher consumption of sugar and saturated fat correlated with heart disease, but were also reflections of a larger, health-harming creature: the modernization of our food system and lifestyle, especially as it related to a nation's affluence. With greater wealth generally came more cars, televisions, and radios—and with them a rapid decline in physical activity. (The twentieth century was the first time in human history where sedentary living could be possible for the masses.)

Sedentary living, we now know, induces rapid changes in how the body handles the food we eat, compromising our insulin sensitivity and glucose tolerance—both factors in conditions ranging from heart disease to diabetes, and influencing our ability to metabolize saturated fat and sugar.

Modernization and wealth, likewise, introduce a slew of "new" foods and non-foods that often replace the traditional cuisine of a population. Meat intake goes up because more people can afford it. Processed vegetable oils enter the scene. Chronic stress, at a level unprecedented in human history, follows the fast-paced jobs of the modern world. Each element is invariably tangled with the rest, woven into a quilt too intricate to disassemble and study in isolated pieces.

If Yudkin and Keys had conceded they each knew only part of the elephant, so to speak, perhaps they would have joined forces and gained a more complete picture of heart disease and other modern ailments. And maybe they would have realized the creature they were chasing was much larger than either of their theories could capture alone.

Nonetheless, history extended its hand toward Keys and hoisted him firmly into the winner's circle. And as the cogs of epidemiology continued to crank, another midcentury project helped keep him there: the Framingham Heart Study, which we're about to explore in the next chapter.

FROM CRETE TO CAMBRIDGE:
THE MEDITERRANEAN DIET, TAKE 2

Professor of medicine. Nutrition chair at Harvard. Author of more than one thousand peer-reviewed articles on diet and disease. Second-most cited researcher in clinical medicine. If there were such thing as a celebrity researcher, Walter Willett—a man who wears all of these hats and then some—would've earned his star on the Hollywood Walk of Fame long ago. Amongst Willett's many gifts to the world is the Harvard Healthy Eating Pyramid, an attempt to repackage the Mediterranean diet with some oily tweaks. (To keep pace with the USDA's food-guide shape upgrade, Harvard more recently released a Healthy Eating Plate as well.)

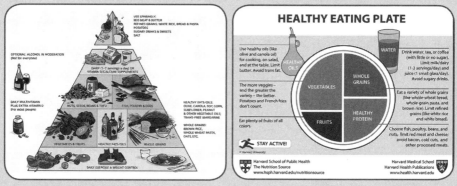

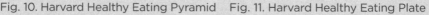

Fig. 10. Harvard Healthy Eating Pyramid   Fig. 11. Harvard Healthy Eating Plate

Like most things sprouting from an Ivy League vine, the Harvard pyramid seems fabulously highbrow and smart—an intelligent revision of the USDA's blunder, with an enticing European spin. And in many ways, it is. Inspired largely by the Cretan Mediterranean diet and championed by Keys, the Harvard pyramid and plate abolishes the food-industry concessions to keep refined starches on the table.

Grains, the superstar of the USDA's pyramid, fill less than half a tier instead of stealing the whole show. A new "base" of daily exercise and weight control emphasizes the importance of non-diet components of health. And to some, the Harvard pyramid's crowning glory is its grand adieu to the lowfat message: it embraces vegetable oils such as olive, canola, soybean, corn, sunflower, and peanut, as well as trans-fat free vegetable margarines. (Animal fats—particularly butter and fatty meats—are still stuffed into the pyramid's "use sparingly" attic.)

Indeed, Willett doesn't mince words when explaining why federal diet advice has largely been a failure. In a 2004 interview with PBS's *Frontline,* he described the USDA's food pyramid as "not compatible with good scientific evidence" and "out of date from the day it was printed," due mainly to its universal condemnation of fat and unscrupulous promotion of starches.[85] Likewise, the Harvard School of Public Health's "Nutrition Source" website notes the USDA's recommendations were "influenced by people with business interests in the messages the icons sent."[86] Harvard's spin on the pyramid and plate, by contrast, "are unaffected by businesses and organizations with a stake in their messages."[87]

By and large, Harvard's pyramid and plate do weed out many of the flaws plaguing the USDA's advice—but they're still far from perfect. Apart from the issue of individual starch tolerance, which we'll hash out in *Herbivore's Dilemma,* one glaring and potentially dangerous issue stands out: the Harvard pyramid's clear endorsement of industrial oils, which contain a level of omega-6 fats unknown to the human body until just the last century.

Willett, a well-known champion of such oils (and whose vocal, pro-omega-6 views don't always mesh with those of other researchers), felt that American heart disease trends are fabulously supportive of the move towards higher polyunsaturated fat (PUFA) intake. In describing the '70s-era dietary advice to replace saturated fat with polyunsaturated fat, Willett claims the subsequent PUFA increase was probably the biggest reason American heart disease rates dropped in the '70s and early '80s.[88] (His observation is a shining example of the "correlation isn't causation" rule: during the same period heart disease mortality began its rapid falloff, cigarette smoking had also entered its decline—throwing some uncertainty on the claim that PUFA intake was really the driving force.[89])

It's important to note that the Harvard pyramid's highly vegetable-oiled base is a theoretical addition rather than a component of any traditional, health-promoting diet of the Mediterranean (or anywhere else, for that matter). While olive oil was certainly a highlight of the menus there, corn oil, soybean oil, cottonseed oil, and other fats requiring heavy industrial processing arrived only in more recent decades. Willett's choice to include them in the pyramid is based largely on their tendency to lower blood cholesterol—though such foods have not, in any decent study, been shown to improve actual mortality rates.

In fact, Israel, a nation with a high prevalence of cardiovascular disease, hypertension, and insulin resistance, is one of the only real-world examples we have of a population consuming high levels of PUFA oils. Their intake is about 8 percent higher than the US, and 10 to 12 percent higher than most of Europe.[90] The apparent disharmony between Israeli health and what conventional wisdom says about a high-PUFA diet has given rise to the term "Israeli Paradox." But as we'll see in the next chapter, there's nothing paradoxical about poor health outcomes following a long and steady intake of industrial vegetable oils.

8
A Little Town in Massachusetts

FRAMINGHAM, MASSACHUSETTS. Population: 68,313. Land area: 25.1 square miles. Home of the New England Wildflower Society, three Starbucks stores, and the single-most influential heart disease study of all time—one that helped brand "cholesterol" as a word to be feared.

The Framingham Heart Study—an ongoing project currently on its third generation—was born out of a quest for discovery. In the 1940s, the US government noted a sudden rise in the occurrence of heart attacks. Lives were being lost en masse, but the reasons why were mystifying. No one had yet identified what was causing this strange new epidemic, much less how to stop it. And like Ancel Keys, the government turned to WWII mortality statistics to help answer some questions.

Framingham thus emerged as an antenna to probe out the dark, foreign world of heart disease. The study would fall under the care of the freshly created National Heart Institute (now expanded into the National Heart, Lung, and Blood Institute). And like the Seven Countries Study, would also become one of our most iconic examples of a *prospective cohort* design—in which investigators follow a core group of people for many years, observing both their lives and their eventual deaths. What better way to understand the nation's burgeoning heart disease epidemic than to round up thousands of seemingly healthy folks, see who gets heart disease and who stays healthy, and then figure out what those two groups were doing differently?

The city—an otherwise uneventful Boston suburb—became the study's launch pad due to its delightful normalcy. Framingham typified Anytown, USA, and it was hoped the study's findings would reach far beyond city limits and have relevance for the nation at large. Plus, the timing was perfect: no longer funding World War

II, the US government could now put money into executing such a mammoth project. The biggest hurdle was finding over five thousand volunteers—about half of the city's adult population—who were willing to get poked, prodded, and surveyed up the wazoo for the study's anticipated two decades, gaining nothing in return except for bragging rights and electrode bruises. It was a risky and expensive venture, one made more complicated by the era's lack of electronic calculators and copy machines and other technological luxuries that help track data today.

But despite an upstream swim, Framingham emerged victorious. In 1948, the study officially commenced. A total of 5,209 men and women had agreed to participate in a project that would soon change the landscape of medicine, forming the study's first cohort and casting the earliest rays of light on the etiology of heart disease.

(Over the years, as the original cohort dwindled, more would be spawned in its wake—including the Offspring Study, which pulled in the grown children (and their spouses) from the first group; and the Third Generation Study, which included the grown grandchildren of the original cohort to explore the genetic threads linking heart disease within families; and finally, two Omni Cohorts, which pulled in ethnic minorities to diversify Framingham's European-dominant population.)

As data from the Framingham Study began to accumulate, so, too, did revolutionary breakthroughs in our understanding of health and disease. The scroll of Framingham's gifts to the world could fill a novel. It was Framingham that gave birth to the term "risk factors," or variables associated with higher rates of a disease—in this case, connecting the correlative dots between heart disease and diabetes, high cholesterol, hypertension, obesity, and sedentary living.

It confirmed the link between smoking and declining heart health. It unveiled the protective effects of high HDL cholesterol.

It served as the first-ever heart disease study to include women. It shattered dangerous myths of a bygone era in medicine—that high blood pressure was helpful for the elderly, that arterial plaque was an inevitable part of aging, that smoking cigarettes was a harmless pastime.

Its scientific publications currently exceed twenty-four thousand and continue to grow annually.

But beyond these, Framingham's most salient contribution to the nutrition world was cementing the lipid hypothesis into scientific consensus. Rising against a backdrop of short-term clinical trials showing saturated fat raises cholesterol, Framingham's finding that higher blood cholesterol levels associate with greater heart disease mortality—landing cholesterol as a front-and-center *risk factor*—seemed to be the ultimate thread sewing saturated fat to the nation's declining health. As its findings dovetailed with those of Keys, Framingham ultimately helped usher America onto its now-well-trodden anti-fat path.

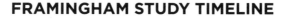

FRAMINGHAM STUDY TIMELINE

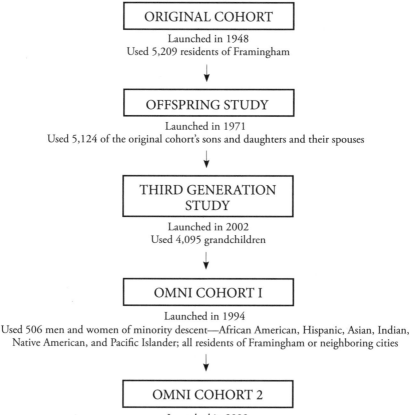

ORIGINAL COHORT

Launched in 1948
Used 5,209 residents of Framingham

OFFSPRING STUDY

Launched in 1971
Used 5,124 of the original cohort's sons and daughters and their spouses

THIRD GENERATION
STUDY

Launched in 2002
Used 4,095 grandchildren

OMNI COHORT I

Launched in 1994
Used 506 men and women of minority descent—African American, Hispanic, Asian, Indian,
Native American, and Pacific Islander; all residents of Framingham or neighboring cities

OMNI COHORT 2

Launched in 2003
Used 410 additional minority participants

Fig. 12.

Less advertised, however, is the fact that **Framingham—with its reams of long-term data on diet and death—failed to show that folks eating more saturated fat were actually getting more heart disease, or even had higher cholesterol levels than their lower-fat kin.** William Castelli, who'd been serving as the study's director since 1979, cited the anomalous finding in a 1992 *Archives of Internal Medicine* editorial. Calling the absence of solid saturated fat-heart disease evidence in cohort studies "disappointing," he wrote:

In Framingham, Massachusetts, the more saturated fat one ate, the more cholesterol one ate, the more calories one ate, the lower people's serum cholesterol ... the opposite of what the equations provided by Hegsted et al and Keys et al would predict.[1]

Although it's become somewhat of a tradition to lift this particular quote out of context and sling it as ammo against the diet-heart hypothesis, there was a bit more to the story. Castelli also maintained that in the case of Framingham, with its data eternally locked in observational limbo, lack of evidence wasn't evidence of lack. Following his oft-quoted statement, which he later remarked was "correct ... but its interpretation [by cholesterol skeptics] wrong," he wrote of his deeper faith in controlled trials to clarify saturated fat's nefarious role:[2]

Eventually, diet intervention trials [that reduced saturated fat] were done, and where the follow-up got out beyond three years, they all show the same thing. The larger the percentage fall in cholesterol, the larger percentage fall in coronary heart disease. In view of this ... those traditional dietary constituents, saturated fat and cholesterol, [are] known to have an adverse effect on blood lipids, and thereby, on the subsequent development of coronary disease end points.[3]

Regardless of Castelli's take on the matter, Framingham's struggle to incriminate saturated fat and cholesterol was noteworthy. His comments in 1992 referred to an early analysis of the data—a lost-in-the-dusty-tomes-of-history report coined the Framingham Diet Study—that asked one of the most pressing questions of the time: *Does diet influence cholesterol and heart disease?*

It was the brainchild of statistician Tavia Gordon, who felt compelled to do something worthwhile with the ocean of food data Framingham had collected. "Unfortunately, these data were never incorporated into a definitive report by the original investigators," Gordon lamented in his paper's editorial note, "and a large amount of very careful and thoughtful work has lain unused in the Framingham files."[4] In an attempt to remedy that, Gordon took it upon himself to prune through the data with his own mathematically deft hands and compile the results into something meaningful.

Based on a sample of nearly a thousand Framingham adults followed between 1957 and 1960, the now-obscure project chased the hypothesis that blood cholesterol and heart disease were linked intimately with dietary factors such as animal fat intake and calorie balance. It was a hypothesis that would eventually win over the scientific world, drive decades of public health policy, and dictate our collective level of postprandial guilt. Yet despite poring over three years of data from Framingham men and women, Gordon's hypothesis hunt—no matter how many statistical spears he wielded—couldn't bring home a single kill.

"No relationship could be discerned within the study cohort between food intake and serum cholesterol level," was the disappointing summary in Gordon's report. **Dietary cholesterol seemed to have no bearing on the participants' wide range of blood cholesterol levels. Nor did the ratio of animal fat to plant fat in the diet. Nor did the total percentage of calories from fat. Nor did protein intake. Nor did carbohydrate intake.**

The one glimmer of significance was a small but present trend among higher-calorie, higher-fat eating men to have lower cholesterol levels than the rest—a finding that was neither powerful enough to raise eyebrows nor supportive of the hypothesis under question. (It was also potentially confounded by the men's exercise habits, with the more physically active of the bunch eating more food in general.)

Gordon's concluding words, all but forgotten today, should haunt those who view Framingham as a nail in saturated fat's coffin.

> There is, in short, no suggestion of any relation between diet and
> the subsequent development of coronary heart disease in the study
> group, despite a distinct elevation of serum cholesterol level in men

developing coronary heart disease.… The data strongly suggest that if there really is any association between diet intake and serum cholesterol level in the Framingham Study population, it is probably a weak one.

In some ways, the earliest years of the study—and Gordon's long-buried analysis of it—may be the most illuminating for all things diet: the American menu hadn't yet busted into a jamboree of processed snacks, high fructose corn syrup, multivarious forms of corn and wheat, lab-concocted flavorings and chemicals, and other sketchy items that only vaguely resemble food. Indeed, all of these may exert their effects on our bodies in ways other than their simple fat or carbohydrate content. With the nation's diet increasing in such confounders, the data gleaned from Framingham's adolescent years is somewhat precious, of a simpler nature nearly impossible to replicate today.

As Framingham chugged forward, more nuanced fat and cholesterol findings began to surface—all adding valuable layers to our knowledge base, but none corroborating the diet-heart hypothesis a growing number of scientists were hanging their hats on. Quite the opposite, a trek through Framingham's jungle of publications does little to paint saturated fat and dietary cholesterol as baneful:

A 1992 analysis found that low intakes of saturated fat and dietary cholesterol were associated with small, dense LDL particles—considered *more* atherogenic than larger particles, due to their ability to rapidly infiltrate artery walls—thus winning saturated fat an unexpected point on the health scoreboard.[5]

A study of Framingham women found food intake utterly unrelated to their blood cholesterol, except for a very weak total-fat-and-blood-cholesterol connection among postmenopausal women only.[6]

Eggs, those tasty but maligned cholesterol bombs, were also off the hook: researchers couldn't find any difference in the blood-cholesterol distribution patterns among egg lovers (eating up to twenty-four per week) and egg avoiders (eating as little as zero per week)—leading to the conclusion that within the Framingham population, "merely avoiding eggs in the diet will have little or no effect on blood cholesterol level."[7]

Among men, only the youngest of the study's participants saw any relationship between fat intake and heart disease, and the link was primarily from *monounsaturated* fat—the kind we've deemed "heart healthy." The association with saturated fat was only marginal, and no fat-and-heart-disease link surfaced at all among the older men.[8]

Even more troubling for the nationwide message to trim down on fat was a discovery about the *other* chief cardiovascular killer: stroke. **By 1997, the study's data was clearly showing that folks eating less saturated fat and total fat were suffering from higher rates of stroke—a pattern previously seen in some Asian populations, but had scarcely been studied among Westerners.**[9] In Framingham, the relationship between lowfat and saturated fat intake and stroke persisted even after adjusting for cigarette smoking, glucose intolerance, body mass index, fruit and vegetable intake, alcohol consumption, cholesterol levels, blood pressure, and other potentially confounding forces.

Even Framingham's findings on blood cholesterol fail to support a universal "the lower the better" recommendation. Among women aged fifty-six to seventy, the lowest mortality rates—both short-term and long-term—emerged when total cholesterol was between 240 and 280 mg/dL, values that would earn an immediate statin prescription in most doctors' offices today.[10] Combined with the fact that cholesterol levels under 240 mg/dL went hand-in-hand with greater mortality for women above seventy years old, the researchers had to conclude that their results "do not support the hypothesis that cholesterol under 200 mg/dL leads to decreased mortality in women over fifty-five years old."[11]

Multiple papers spawned by Framingham also link low cholesterol levels with greater risk of cancer, even after accounting for the possibility of cholesterol reduction being a product rather than a cause of early-stage cancer.[12] One analysis found that men with both low cholesterol levels and obesity were four times as likely to develop colon cancer than men with average cholesterol and weight.[13]

And for those valuing their brainpower, low cholesterol turned out to be a startling bummer: a 2005 analysis found that folks with the lowest total cholesterol—even in "desirable" ranges up to 200 mg/dL—scored the worst on measures of verbal fluency, attention, concentration, abstract reasoning, and a composite score for multiple cognitive domains.[14] Those with higher cholesterol, on the other hand, exhibited strikingly better cognitive performance.

While Framingham certainly deserves some blazing candles in the Landmark Study Shrine for its findings on smoking, diabetes, blood pressure, physical activity, genetics, and other risk factors for heart disease, it dredged up little to suggest saturated fat is a threat to heart health—or even support our current cholesterol targets and the statin prescribing practices that come along with them. It was a study whose reputation didn't match its reality, and whose findings have suffered in the hands of profitable drug industries and a biased scientific climate.

By now, you can see how the early heart-disease studies failed to show a cause-and-effect relationship between dietary fat and heart disease. But what happens when the diet-heart hypothesis is put to the test in a way that *could* determine cause and effect?

In the next chapter, we'll explore the clinical trials that set out to swap animal fat for polyunsaturated vegetable oils—a maneuver still recommended by the USDA and other health organizations today.

Their findings may surprise you.

RESEARCH MILESTONES

1960　Cigarette smoking found to increase the risk of heart disease

1961　Cholesterol level, blood pressure, and electrocardiogram abnormalities found to increase the risk of heart disease

1967　Physical activity found to reduce the risk of heart disease and obesity to increase the risk of heart disease

1970　High blood pressure found to increase the risk of stroke

1970　Atrial fibrillation increases stroke risk 5-fold

1976　Menopause found to increase the risk of heart disease

1978　Psychosocial factors found to affect heart disease

1988　High levels of HDL cholesterol found to reduce risk of death

1994　Enlarged left ventricle (one of two lower chambers of the heart) shown to increase the risk of stroke

1996　Progression from hypertension to heart failure described

1998　Framingham Heart Study researchers identify that atrial fibrillation is associated with an increased risk of all-cause mortality

1998　Development of simple coronary disease prediction algorithm involving risk factor categories to allow physicians to predict multivariate coronary heart disease risk in patients without overt CHD

1999　Lifetime risk at age 40 years of developing coronary heart disease is one in two for men and one in three for women

2001　High-normal blood pressure is associated with an increased risk of cardiovascular disease, emphasizing the need to determine whether lowering high-normal blood pressure can reduce the risk of cardiovascular disease

2002　Lifetime risk of developing high blood pressure in middle-aged adults is 9 in 10

2002　Obesity is a risk factor for heart failure

2004　Serum aldosterone levels predict future risk of hypertension in non-hypertensive individuals

2005　Lifetime risk of becoming overweight exceeds 70 percent, that for obesity approximates 1 in 2

2006　The National Heart, Lung, and Blood Institute (NHLBI) of the National Institutes of Health announces a new genome-wide association study at the Framingham Heart Study in collaboration with Boston University School of Medicine to be known as the SHARe project (SNP Health Association Resource)

2007   Based on evaluation of a densely interconnected social network of 12,067 people assessed as part of the Framingham Heart Study, network phenomena appear to be relevant to the biologic and behavioral trait of obesity, and obesity appears to spread through social ties

2008   Based on analysis of a social network of 12,067 people participating in the Framingham Heart Study, researchers discover that social networks exert key influences on decision to quit smoking

2008   Discovery by Framingham Heart Study and publication of four risk factors that raise probability of developing precursor of heart failure; new 30-year risk estimates developed for serious cardiac events

2009   Framingham Heart Study cited by the American Heart Association among the top 10 cardiovascular research achievements of 2009, "Genome-wide Association Study of Blood Pressure and Hypertension: Genome-wide association study identifies eight loci associated with blood pressure"

2009   A new genetic variant associated with increased susceptibility for atrial fibrillation, a prominent risk factor for stroke and heart failure, is reported in two studies based on data from the Framingham Heart Study

2009   Framingham Heart Study researchers find parental dementia may lead to poor memory in middle-aged adults.

2009   Framingham Heart Study researchers find high leptin levels may protect against Alzheimer's disease and dementia

2010   Sleep apnea tied to increased risk of stroke

2010   Framingham Heart Study researchers identify additional genes that may play a role in Alzheimer's disease

2010   Framingham Heart Study finds fat around the abdomen associated with smaller, older brains in middle-aged adults

2010   Framingham Heart Study finds genes link puberty timing and body fat in women

2010   Having first-degree relative with atrial fibrillation associated with increased risk for this disorder

2009 -2010   Framingham Heart Study researchers contribute to discovering hundreds of new genes underlying major heart disease risk factors—body mass index, blood cholesterol, cigarette smoking, blood pressure and glucose/diabetes

2010   First definitive evidence that occurrence of stroke by age 65 years in a parent increased risk of stroke in offspring by 3-fold

9
PUFA-rama:
The Rise of Vegetable Oils

THE YEAR WAS 1837, and the place was Cincinnati—the nation's hub for all things pig. With its prime location, explosion of tanneries and slaughterhouses, and herds of swine tottering through the streets, the city had earned the nickname "Porkopolis," shipping pork galore down river and feeding mouths near and far. And for two of the city's accidental transplants—William Procter and James Gamble—that meant a steady supply of their business's most precious commodity: lard.

But cooking with it was the last thing on the men's minds. Instead, the rendered fat was the chief ingredient for their candles and soaps.

That the men had met at all—much less launched the now-largest consumer goods company in the world—was somewhat serendipitous. Procter, an English candle maker, had been voyaging to the great American West when his first wife died of cholera—cutting short his travels and leaving him stuck in Cincinnati. Gamble, an Irish soap maker, had been Illinois-bound when unexpected illness plopped him in the Queen City as well. Cupid must've seen a prime opportunity for meddling, because the men ended up falling in love with two Cincinnati women who just happened to be sisters. Marriage ensued, and with it came their new father-in-law's flash of insight that the men, who were already competing for the same materials for their soap and candle-making pursuits, ought to become business partners.[1]

And thus was born Procter and Gamble—or P&G, as we know it today.

The Death of Lard

Though Procter & Gamble enjoyed early success, its lifeblood—the animal-fat industry—saw the first hint of its eventual undoing near the turn of the century. It was a death-march summoned largely by journalist Upton Sinclair. After a two-month investigation of Chicago's meatpacking district, he penned a fictional tale inspired by the horrors he'd witnessed: revolting conditions for immigrant workers, unsanitary meat-handling practices, and an utter abuse of power by the nation's "industrial masters." It wasn't long before the novel, titled *The Jungle* and first published as serial installments in the socialist newspaper *Appeal to Reason*, took the nation by storm.

Unfortunately, it wasn't the kind of storm Sinclair was banking on. While he assumed the book would evoke sympathy for the working class (and, if all went as planned, win support for the socialist movement), readers were too shocked by his descriptions of meat production to care much about the workers' social plight: the stench of the killing beds, the acid-devoured fingers of pickle-room men, the poisoned rats scrambling onto meat piles and inadvertently joining America's food supply. If nothing else, Sinclair succeeded in churning an unprecedented number of stomachs. And the sinking ship of meat's reputation brought with it another casualty: lard. As one gruesome passage described:

> The other men, who worked in the tank rooms full of steam, and in some of which there were open vats near the level of the floor, their peculiar trouble was that they fell into the vats; and when they were fished out, there was never enough of them to be worth exhibiting—sometimes they would be overlooked for days, till all but the bones of them had gone out to the world as Durham's Pure Leaf Lard![2]

The image of lard containing the renderings of *people* proved too vivid to purge from memory—a sort of Soylent Green prelude. Shortly after *The Jungle* exploded onto the scene, sales of American meat products sank by half.[3] And while the book never elicited the political response Sinclair had hoped for, it did lead to a food-safety uproar so profound that the US government had to step in and calm its horrified citizens. In 1906, mere months after the book's debut, Congress passed two landmark acts—the Federal Meat Inspection Act and the Pure Food and Drug Act of 1906—to enforce standards for food production and help Americans feel better about what they were eating. (The two acts collectively set the groundwork for the Food and Drug Administration years later.)

Believing *The Jungle* failed as a social commentary but inadvertently succeeded as an exposé on food sanitation, Sinclair later remarked: "I aimed at the public's heart, and by accident I hit it in the stomach!"[4]

But even if Sinclair's book managed to sour Americans on lard, no alternatives other than butter currently existed to satisfy the country's cooking needs. At least not yet.

Over in France, chemist Paul Sabatier had been busily developing the *hydrogenation* process—the act of shooting hydrogen atoms into an unsaturated chemical compound. Though his early work was limited to vapors, it wasn't long before another scientist, Wilhelm Normann, replicated the procedure using oils—demonstrating for the first time that a liquid fat could, through deft chemical tweaking, become solid at room temperature. At the time, it seemed on par with lead-to-gold alchemy.

And best of all, the thick, creamy result of hydrogenation was exactly what P&G needed to seal their legacy. Although the company spent years oblivious to those oversea hydrogenation miracles, a pivotal moment came in 1907 when Edwin Kayser—a recent transplant to Cincinnati, and chemist for the company that owned the rights to the process of hydrogenating oil—approached Procter & Gamble's business manager with an idea.[5] Why not use this revolutionary new substance to make soap?

It didn't take long before the dream was a reality. By 1908, the company owned eight cottonseed mills and had secured a steady supply of the oil they needed to feed production.

Elbows-deep in the cottonseed market, Procter & Gamble realized their soap making—as lucrative as it was—had only tapped the surface of cottonseed oil's potential. And the company soon found itself facing a new conundrum: the dawn of the electrical age. Although it would be many more years before the whole country was firelessly alight, candle sales were already taking a blow, and Procter and Gamble knew they needed to keep pace with the changing world to avoid a financial nosedive. It was time to enter the kitchen.

The Birth of Trans Fats

In 1910, Procter & Gamble applied for a US patent on the use of hydrogenation for making a human-grade food product. Compared to the flowery, rhetorically brilliant hype it would later receive, the description was cool and clinical:

> This invention is a food product consisting of a vegetable oil, pref-erably cottonseed oil, partially hydrogenated, and hardened to a homogenous white or yellowish semi-solid closely resembling lard. The special object of the invention is to provide a new food product for a shortening in cooking.[6]

After a few failed attempts to claim a name—"Krispo" was taken by a cracker company; "Cryst" sounded religious—Procter and Gamble settled on "Crisco," derived from "crystallized cottonseed oil."[7] The name would quite literally become a household term.

Up until that point, a handful of processed vegetable oils had presence in America—but unlike today, their claim to fame had nothing to do with being edible. In fact, stomachs were often the *last* place highly refined oils would end up. Peanut oil had gained some publicity as a potential fuel: one company managed to coax a small diesel engine into running on it during the 1900 Paris Exhibition.[8] And cottonseed oil made its American debut back in 1768, when a Pennsylvania doctor figured out how to collect the fat from crushed cottonseeds—which he then used as a treatment for colic.[9] (Woe be to his patients, that crude oil was teeming with *gossypol*—a chemical that causes infertility, low blood potassium, and sometimes paralysis, and can only be removed from cottonseeds through heavy processing.[10])

Ginning mills were thrilled someone wanted to haul away their cottonseed. Through much of the 1800s, the stuff had simply been left to rot in gin houses, or occasionally dumped illegally into rivers. But one man's trash had become another man's treasure, so to speak, and P&G had pioneered what's now an American tradition: getting rid of agricultural waste products by feeding them to humans. The company had effectively bridged the gap between garbage and food.

By 1911, Crisco made its official debut. And what a debut it was. Almost immediately, the new fat had gained not only the nation's trust, but also its passionate love. Within a year, over 2.5 million pounds of Crisco had flown off the shelves; by 1916, that number reached sixty million.[11]

How could a single product dominate the cooking world at warp speed—rising from total obscurity into an indispensible staple in a matter of months? P&G had a back-patting answer for themselves: that housewives, chefs, doctors, and dieticians "were glad to be shown a product which at once would make for more *digestible* foods, more *economical* foods, and better *tasting* foods." Crisco exploded onto the scene all on its own, was the implication. It was just *that* good!

In reality, though, Crisco's expedited fame was owed mainly to some of the most skillful, manipulative ad campaigns the young century had seen. Knowing it would be hard to convince housewives—the gatekeepers of America's kitchens—to give up their familiar lard and butter in exchange for this strange new item, P&G had hyped their product like few things had ever been hyped before. The company mailed samples to fifteen thousand grocers in America. Thousands of flyers were circulated among jobbers.[12] The company deftly played upon women's burning desire to be "modern," persuading them that clinging to animal fats in the face of this new scientific discovery would be akin to their grandmothers refusing to give up the spinning wheel.[13]

But most powerful of all was *The Story of Crisco*—equal parts advertisement and cookbook—which P&G handed out to housewives free of charge. Its 615 recipes, all united by their shared ingredient, Crisco, ranged from tantalizing (Clear Almond Taffy; Snow Pudding with Custard) to whimsical (Calf's Head Vinaigrette; Mushrooms Cooked Under Glass Bells). The true marketing genius, however, came from the book's introductory chapters. Carefully grooming readers into future Crisco acolytes, the book first painted animal fats in the most dismal light possible, expounding their "objectionable features" and whetting appetites for a better replacement. Crisco was presented as a panacea of sorts—healthier than lard, more economical than butter, and altogether in a category of its own. Everything other fats did wrong, Crisco did right. P&G managed to create a demand for something people hadn't even known they wanted.

(As a peek into the different meat world of the day, the book was also busting with recipes for ox tongue, baked brains, heart, kidney omelets, sweetbreads (that's the more appetizing term for pancreas or thymus), stewed liver, and tripe (the rubbery lining of ruminant stomachs)—all foods fit for an impressive supper back in the day. As we'll see in the upcoming *Meet Your Meat* chapter, the systematic purging of these foods from the modern menu has done us a great nutritional disservice.)

In the wake of the grungy, repulsive world of meatpacking depicted in *The Jungle*, Crisco built its image on purity. Its factories were gleaming, sterile wonderlands. Its product was bright as snow. Its packaging included not only a tin can, but also an over-wrap of white paper, emphasizing its pristine state. Everything about the product screamed *undefiled*. Like the incorruptible relics of a saint, Crisco seemed eternally taintless—exactly what America, eager to wipe itself of the grime of the 1800s and enter a cleaner century, was hungry for.

Incidentally, *The Story of Crisco* also captured a fascinating view of fat from the early 1900s—a perspective that would face extinction once the USDA unleashed its smack down on all things lipid. In its chapter titled "Man's Most Important Food, Fat," *The Story of Crisco* remarked, "No other food supplies our bodies with the *drive*, the vigor, which fat gives. No other food has been given so little study in proportion to its importance." (Emphasis in original.)

Back in the day, Crisco was indeed nothing short of a miracle. It came from plants; it was firm; it was tasty; it was cheap; it fried foods without smoking; and huzzah, it was even kosher and *parava*—usable with both milk and meat per Jewish dietary law. (Rabbi Margolies of New York, who was in charge of approving the food's kosher label, remarked "the Hebrew Race had been waiting four thousand years for Crisco."[14])

It wasn't long before this new dietary messiah had infiltrated pantries, fryers, cakes, pies, omelets, meatloaves, and the very heart of America's psyche. During World War II, butter rationing helped push Crisco and margarine to center stage, and oils from corn and soybean joined cottonseed oil as the slippery darlings of a new food technology. It wasn't long before science seemed to be cheering on the trend as well.

In 1961, with the famous Ancel Keys now an iron-jawed board member, the American Heart Association (AHA) officially threw its weight behind the idea that saturated fat was causing heart disease— implying that P&G's profit-driven corralling of Americans away from lard and butter had accidentally been good for their health. Around the same year, the nation's margarine consumption exceeded butter intake for the first time in history.[15]

It seemed Crisco had done the impossible and lived up to its own unbridled hype. But there was a dark side to all this purity. With cottonseed oil's omega-6 to omega-3 ratio registering a magnitude 258 to 1, Crisco became the first ingredient to unleash unprecedented levels of linoleic acid—a polyunsaturated fat—into the American diet. Unknown to even the sharpest nutritionists of the day, Crisco had invited two killers into the American diet: trans fat resulting from partially hydrogenating oils and an astronomical intake of omega-6 fats—both now known to increase the risk of heart disease and cause inflammatory immune responses. It would be many decades before anyone realized what had gone so horribly wrong. In fact, the USDA would promote trans fats all the way up until 2005.

But long before then, there had been growing suspicion that trans fats were fatal to our well-being. As early as the 1950s, while Ancel Keys was busy winning the world over to Team Anti-Saturated Fat, other researchers were noting the uncanny connection between the use of partially hydrogenated oils (and the trans fat they contained) and the rising rates of both heart disease and cancer.[16] While correlation between the two couldn't prove causation any more than Keys's population data could conclusively damn saturated fat, the parallel between trans fat intake and chronic disease rates were beginning to ring some warning bells.

Early research also suggested something awry about trans fats. By the 1960s, scientists realized that while vegetable oils were known to reduce cholesterol levels in controlled trials, the hydrogenated forms of those same oils failed to follow suit. In 1968, it was disconcerting enough for the American Heart Association (AHA) to take note and warn the public in a brochure titled *Diet and Heart Disease*:

> Partial hydrogenation of polyunsaturated fats results in the formation of *trans* forms which are less effective than *cis* forms in lowering cholesterol concentration. It should be noted that many currently available shortenings and margarines are partially hydrogenated and may contain little polyunsaturated fat of the natural *cis,cis* form.[17]

(*Cis* is a chemistry term meaning "on this side," in this case refer-ring to the configuration of atoms in unsaturated fat.)

Despite fifteen thousand pamphlets going to print with a carefully worded demotion of trans fats, none of them would see the light of day. That's because Fred Mattson—a researcher gainfully employed by P&G—convinced the AHA's medical director to remove all traces of those incriminating statements.[18] Instead of distributing the thou-sands of copies they'd already printed, the AHA revised the brochure to make it more palatable to the margarine and shortening industries. Decades would pass before the AHA dragged trans fats back onto the cutting block—years where countless lives were no doubt injured by ignorance of its dangers.

Gag Order on Trans Fats

Remember our conversation back in chapter two on Luise Light, the former USDA nutritionist whose plans for a new food guide—one that would have cracked down on processed starches and sugars in favor of fresh, whole foods—had been so brutally mutated? As it hap-pens, her shadowy safari through the agriculture department included a peek into the era's trans fat research. And what she saw was shocking.

According to Light, the experts she'd convened while developing her food guide in the late seventies were already leery of trans fats—pushing for more research and expressing concern that the partially hydrogenated oils seeping into America's food supply could be quite dangerous.[19] At the same time, scientists at the University of Mary-land were finishing up some intensive research on the impact of trans fats on heart disease. Their findings appeared so incriminating for the lab-created substance that it spurred the USDA to run an analysis of the margarines currently on the market, testing them for their trans fats levels—an endeavor other researchers across the globe were also gaining interest in at the time.[20]

The results were grim. It turned out that the margarine market was a virtual sea of trans fats, with nearly every brand, both regular and those promoted for health, containing disturbingly high levels. According to Light, the head of the USDA's fats lab—who'd spear-headed the analysis—had attempted to spread the findings to other scientists and the public, only to have his efforts thwarted by the steely fist of the USDA. As she described the sorry scene:

The head of the fats lab told me that when he attempted to publish a paper with his findings in a peer-reviewed scientific journal … [the] USDA suppressed it, refusing to allow the information to be published. This eminent, world-renowned scientist told me, with tears in his eyes, that in his twenty-year career in research, he had never been confronted with such blatant political interference in science.[21]

As disturbing as that interference was, it was hardly surprising. Partially hydrogenated oils were a sacred cow for food manufacturers: they were cheaper than animal fats, had a gloriously high melting point, prolonged the shelf life of whatever they touched, and provided just the right consistency to make foods profitably addictive. That Father USDA had rushed in to protect the food industry's favorite commodity wasn't anything new—just business as usual.

(The head of the fats lab, Light described, was so disheartened by corporate interfering that he quit his job to head the nutrition research department at a nearby university.)

Not until 2006 did the FDA officially require food manufacturers to list the trans fat content of their products on nutrition labels. The AHA also dragged its feet until 2006, when it finally advised Americans to cut back on the harmful substance.[22]

But until then, the evidence against trans fat continued to mount. In 1990s, a fresh nugget of research shook up both the scientific community and the public. The study—a well-designed randomized, controlled trial—had taken a group of healthy adults and put them on a series of three different diets, identical in all ways except fat proportion: one high in monounsaturated fat; one high in saturated fat; and one high in trans fats derived from sunflower oil.[23]

During the participants' trans-fat-diet phase, LDL rose while HDL dropped significantly—creating the most unfavorable lipid profile out of any of the diets, and opening a highly probable door for heart disease. While calling for more research to clarify their findings, the researchers concluded: "it would seem prudent for patients at an increased risk of atherosclerosis to avoid a high intake of trans fatty acids."

Nonetheless, the only type of fat continuing to fall under the USDA's sledgehammer was saturated. Despite the results of the 1990 study and other growing concerns about the impact of trans fats on human health, the 1992 food pyramid—and its accompanying pamphlet—didn't even mention the words "trans fat," much less warn that the substance was under investigation as a potential health hazard.

The food pyramid's pamphlet—beneath the heading "Are some types of fat worse than others?"—stated only to limit saturated fat to less than 10 percent of total calories because it could raise cholesterol and cause heart disease. Absent were any caveats for other fat-based dietary components. And worse, the pamphlet specifically advised consumers to tilt their fat choices toward margarines with "vegetable oil" listed as their first ingredient, effectively steering folks toward some of the richest sources of trans fat in existence.[24]

Curiously enough, up until the 1992 Food Guide Pyramid, the USDA was probably the most lax of all the official organizations when it came to replacing animal fats with high-omega-6 oils and partially hydrogenated fats. But then again, in a theme still repeated today, public health recommendations were virtually the last to respond to advancing science—plodding along as slow, cautious, lumbering beasts chronically out of pace with the latest discoveries in nutrition.

With the trans fat hoopla brewing in the background, the showdown between saturated fat and polyunsaturated was stealing a far more public spotlight. Recall last chapter's discussion on the Seven Countries Study. Keys had barely concluded its first follow-up when long-term trials were beginning to show that the diet-heart hypothesis borne at the population level didn't always pan out in controlled settings.

But as often happens when a nutritional theory enters the echo chamber of mainstream belief, the results of those studies were squeezed, bent, and shoddily interpreted in order to bolster the anti-saturated-fat movement of the time. Several of the most important trials—whose innards we're about to explore—suggested that cholesterol-lowering diets, stuffed full of "heart healthy" vegetable oils, were actually *increasing* total mortality, cancer rates, and even heart disease itself, despite being cited as evidence for the contrary. It was a reality swept out of sight by ideological forces and groupthink.

Let's now take a look at what *really* went on behind the scenes of our most prominent diet-heart trials, and why the nation's lust for vegetable oil —both then and now—has likely done more harm than good.

The Finnish Mental Hospital Trial

If ever a trophy study existed, the Finnish Mental Hospital Trial is certainly it. With over 750 peer-reviewed citations between its two main publications, the trial became one of the most influential and widely referenced studies of its kind, laying the foundation for widespread polyunsaturaed fat (PUFA) consumption. Even today, the study fuels meta-analyses, literature reviews, and scientific debates on the merits of saturated fat and PUFAs. Along with locking Keys posthumously in the scientific winner's circle, it shaped a great deal of the nutritional recommendations still ringing in our ears today.

Yet the trial isn't noteworthy because of its meticulous design. Or its tight control of variables. Or its uncontestable confirmation of the hypothesis it set out to test. It's noteworthy because it failed on virtually every account and catapulted to fame anyway.

We'll get back to that in a minute. But first, some background.

As you may recall, the famous Keys did a bang-up job exposing the scientific community to his diet-heart hypothesis back in the late 1950s. And once the skepticism died down, other researchers opened to the possibility that saturated fat could indeed be driving the world's sudden rash of heart disease.

There was just one problem. No one had completed any long-term trials testing on whether swapping saturated animal fats for PUFA-rich oils would actually protect against heart disease in a measurable, verifiable, objective way. Such trials, it was reasoned, would be the dot-connecter between the existing observational and experimental evidence—but until they were conducted, too many question marks remained. Would controlled human studies unfold in the same direction as observational ones? Would a diet-induced slash in blood cholesterol actually keep heart disease at bay? Would saturated fat's fingerprints be causally and conclusively scattered across the scene of the crime?

The time was ripe for some testing. And the Finnish Mental Hospital Trial was one of the first to rise to the challenge. While planning their research venture in 1958, the study's investigators were perfectly clear about their intent: to test whether a cholesterol-reducing diet, low in saturated fat and high in PUFA, could slash heart disease rates.[25] More specifically, the aim was to conduct a *primary prevention* trial— that is, prevent a disease from striking rather than treat or cure one already there. For that reason, the researchers systematically excluded folks with pre-existing heart disease, rounding up only healthy folks, about thirteen thousand middle-aged men and women from two mental hospitals close to Helsinki, to endure twelve years of dietary guinea pigging.

The setup was simple enough. For the first half of the study, one hospital—whose residents effectively acted as the *control group*—received the typical Finnish fare, one rich in saturated dairy fat and scant on vegetable oils.

For those same six years, a different hospital housed the study's *experimental group*—serving the modified, cholesterol-busting menu theorized to combat heart disease: "soft" margarine replaced "hard" margarine and butter. A depressing mix of soybean oil and skim milk replaced whole milk. And any remaining sources of dairy fat were switched out for polyunsaturated lookalikes.

> **Science-jargon reminder:** *secondary prevention* is a form of intervention that happens after an illness (or major risk factor) has already emerged. Unlike *primary prevention,* which focuses on keeping healthy people from succumbing to disease in the first place, *secondary prevention* aims to stop or slow down the progression of a disease that's already reared its ugly head.

And so it went for six years: the control group in one hospital enjoyed plenty of high-fat dairy (and, consequently, saturated fat), while the experimental group in the second hospital consumed a high PUFA menu designed to hammer down blood cholesterol levels.

Then came the great switcheroo.

At the six-year mark, the first hospital replaced its dairy-fat-rich diet with the high PUFA menu, while the second hospital replaced its high PUFA menu with the dairy-fat-rich diet. This leg of the study lasted another six years. (In Science-ese, this is called a *crossover design*—where at a designated point in a study, the control and experimental groups swap what they're doing. Although that's a perfectly fine setup for some trials, it happened to be a fatal flaw for this one—and we'll talk about why in a minute.) When it was Swap O'Clock, the researchers also initiated a "rejuvenation of cohorts," where some younger patients were reeled in to replace the oldest ones—a maneuver to help keep age ranges equal throughout all periods of the study.

Otherwise, the post-switcheroo control and experimental groups would both be six years older than during the first leg of the study.

On the surface, it looked like the researchers had pulled off exactly what they'd set out to do. Some number-crunching confirmed that the high PUFA menu successfully snipped dairy fat out of the equation—dropping it from 22 percent of total fat calories in the "standard Finnish" control diet to only 4 percent in the high PUFA diet. Likewise, the high PUFA diet averaged 68 percent of its fat calories from vegetable oils in "filled milk," soft margarine, and straight-up soybean oil; by contrast, only 9 percent of fat calories came from vegetable oils in the control diet. (It's worth noting, however, that those analyses were averages, and measured only the food each hospital *provided*—not the food the participants actually consumed from that selection.)

For those eager to vilify saturated fat, the trial's results were a thing of much glory. Compared to the control-diet periods, the high PUFA periods triggered a hefty drop in total cholesterol—an average reduction of 12.8 percent for women and 15.5 percent for men.

More important, though, was the high PUFA diet's association with heart health, at least for the study's XY-chromosome crowd. While women didn't see much benefit from PUFA loading in terms of cardiovascular outcomes, the men saw a whopping 44 percent decrease in their incidence of cardiovascular disease when they were eating a low-dairy-fat, high-vegetable-oil cuisine.

Yet amid the confetti-tossing and kazoo-blowing for what appeared to be a victory for the diet-heart hypothesis, a shadow lurked. An army of shadows, in fact—cast by the study's unprecedented legion of flaws. Ultimately, the study was less a "win" for the diet-heart hypothesis and more a "fail" for the scientific method. For starters, turning a critical eye to the Finnish Mental Hospital Trial's fine print, we can see the following:

- The study's *crossover design* made it impossible to actually link the patients' diets with their health outcomes. Because heart disease takes so long to develop, you can't necessarily blame a heart attack on what a person's been eating for the last few months—or even year—when they were eating quite differently for decades prior.

A WORD ON "CROSSING OVER"

Crossover studies have the potential to be seriously abused, especially when it comes to determining the effects of diet on long-term diseases. Let's take a moment to see how.

Imagine living in some parallel universe where your diet consists of nothing but Chicken McNuggets, curly fries, and as many Mountain Dew refills as you can humanly stomach. Now imagine getting diagnosed with scurvy. Spurred to take charge of your health, you swap the Mountain Dew for vitamin-rich orange juice and continue on your merry way.

A year later, you're in the ER with chest pains.

Following the logic set forth by the Finnish Mental Hospital Trial, we'd be tempted to blame the appearance of a new ailment—heart disease, in this case—on the one thing that changed: your beverage of choice. But from the standpoint of disease etiology, that assumption would be a pretty lousy one.

Given how long it takes heart disease to progress before symptoms become obvious, there's no way to know whether it was from that strategic addition of orange juice or the consequence of eating a truly wretched diet for years beforehand. Did the beverage switch trigger heart woes? Or did the previous diet quietly do the bulk of the damage, setting the stage for heart disease that only reached critical mass later on?

The moral of the story is that crossover studies are a terrible way to examine chronic diseases that are years (even decades) in the making. Unlike medications or weight-loss programs whose effects are intentionally rapid, diets aimed at preventing diseases with long incubation periods are tough to study using this type of design.

- The crossover design featured no *washout period* separating each leg of the study. Crossover trials typically force participants to take a breather before they're swapped into a different experimental or control group—a strategy to ensure the effects of one phase of the study don't bleed over into the next one and confound the results. (When that happens, it's called a *carry-over effect.*)

- The study didn't feature adequate *blinding*—an important bias-obliterating tactic for intervention trials. The doctors knew which patients were in the experimental group and which were in the control group at all times, introducing the potential for *diagnostic bias,* where doctors' expectations sway how they interact with and diagnose their patients.

- The *come-and-go residency* in the hospitals made it remarkably difficult to keep the patients' diets consistent. Although folks in each leg of the study were enrolled for up to six years, the amount of time they actually spent in the hospital, receiving the experimental or control diet, could be as low as *six months*— with the remaining time spent eating whatever the heck they wanted at home.

And those weren't the only pitfalls. Along with multiple design flaws, the Finnish Mental Hospital Trial left a few critical variables flapping in the wind, woefully uncontrolled. Let's take a look at what the study detailed in its 1979 publication:

- When each hospital introduced the high PUFA menu, omega-3 intake nearly *tripled* over the standard Finnish diet. Regardless of saturated fat consumption, omega-3 fats have a well-established role in maintaining a healthy heart.[26] It's possible a great deal of the high PUFA diet's benefits came from increasing omega-3 intake rather than cutting out dairy fat.

- This study didn't categorically replace saturated fat with PUFA; it specifically replaced *dairy* fat with soybean oil. That makes it difficult to extrapolate the study's results to all high-saturated fat foods and all PUFA-rich oils. Compared to other sources of saturated animal fat, dairy has a rather unique fatty acid profile—skewed heavily toward palmitic and myristic acids, which tend to raise total cholesterol (especially from LDL) more than other saturated fatty acids.[27, 28] Likewise, soybean oil is much higher in omega-3 fat compared to almost all other vegetable oils—including corn oil, cottonseed oil, safflower oil, sunflower oil, peanut oil, and sesame oil, which are virtually devoid of omega-3. (Soy's linolenic acid content accounts for the omega-3 hike. See sidebar 176 to learn more about omega 3:6 ratios in various oils.)

- Trans fat intake was, on average, *thirteen times higher* in the control groups than in the high PUFA diet groups.[29] As we saw earlier in this chapter, that alone could be responsible for some major heart harm—adding a major handicap to the high-dairy-fat diet periods.

- Between the first and second leg of the study, sugar consumption differed by nearly 50 percent. Total fat intake, too, varied by up to 26 percent between diet periods, and total carbohydrate intake varied by up to 17 percent. The lack of a truly "controlled" status regarding sugar intake and other important variables was enough to spur an editorial from researchers John Rivers and John Yudkin, who criticized the study's design and execution. (The lead author of the Finnish trial responded by acknowledging that the "variations in sugar intake were, of course, regrettable" since "the hospitals, for practical reasons, had to be granted certain freedom in dietary matters."[30])

- And in case the above problems aren't bad enough, the study suffered from one more fatal flaw: the use of Thioridazine—an antipsychotic drug famously known for causing heart problems. (Although Thioridazine was once one of the most popular medications for treating mental disorders, it's now more of a "last resort" drug thanks to its tendency to trigger heart arrhythmia and sudden death.[31]) At the time the Finnish Mental Hospital Trial was conducted,

Thioridazine was in widespread use, and its doses and pre-scription (along with that of other antipsychotics) varied dramatically between hospitals as well as between diet peri-ods. (Indeed, a cardiotoxic drug is not a wise variable to leave uncontrolled during a study of heart disease mortality.)

In short, the Finnish Mental Hospital Trial is a classic case of study gone bad. Of course, controlling people's food intake for years at a time is no easy task—and the study's investigators likely did the best they could with a tricky situation. In that sense, the study's biggest problem *isn't* that it's imperfect, but rather, that it parades hopelessly under a banner of false advertising.

Among its many uncontrolled variables, wobbly design, lack of blinding, and multiple confounders, the study would've been ripped to shreds by the scientific community had it not played such an integral role in getting the diet-heart hypothesis off the ground. In fact, thanks to its dramatic pro-PUFA findings, it remains one of the most supportive trials ever conducted of that hypothesis—making it a shoe-in for meta-analyses and review papers supporting a link between saturated fat, dietary cholesterol, and heart disease.

Oslo Diet-Heart Study

Even if the Finnish Mental Hospital Trial magically disappeared from our repertoire of studies, a second trial—another Nordic nugget—might slide into its spotlighted place: the Oslo Diet-Heart Study. First published as a doctoral thesis in 1966 with follow-up publications in 1968 and 1970, this study is, like its Finnish brother, widely cited as evidence that replacing saturated fat with PUFA-rich vegetable oils does a body good. [32]

But as we shall soon see, this trial has a serious case of mistaken identity. Aiming for *secondary prevention,* the study's lead researcher, Paul Leren, set out to see if an intensive cholesterol-lowering diet could reverse heart disease. He enlisted 412 middle-aged men who'd previously suffered from a heart attack into the study, and randomized them into two groups: a control group who continued to eat their normal diets and an experimental group who were assigned a diet rich in vegetable oil, low in animal fats, and nearly void of dietary choles-terol. As might be expected, the experimental group's PUFA intake skyrocketed to about 20 percent of total energy at the expense of saturated fat.[33] And for five years starting in 1956, the men noshed away as directed.

At first glance, the high PUFA diet seemed to dazzle on the heart disease front. Along with slashing the experimental group's total cholesterol by an average of 17.6 percent, the group suffered only ten fatal heart attacks during the study's five-year run—compared to the control group's twenty-three.

FACTOID: It should be noted that only 4 percent of the study's participants provided any dietary data to be analyzed—and the controls provided a big fat zero. So, we know what the two groups were told to eat, but that might not be the same as what they actually did.

With that in mind, it's no mystery why the Oslo study gets whipped out whenever the diet-heart hypothesis needs some cheerleading. On the surface, it looks like mighty fine evidence for swapping animal fats for vegetable oils.

But the study's first write-up from 1966 reveals that the animal fat-vegetable oil swap was only the caboose in a much longer train of diet modifications. Let's take a look at that original dissertation and see what this study really entailed.

As far as the control group went, there aren't many bones to pick: the folks assigned to this group needed only to carry on with the standard, high-fat Norwegian diet of the time, with no guidelines or restrictions to heed. The only "new" thing in their bellies was a daily multivitamin, which all participants in the trial—whether control or experimental—received.

The high PUFA diet group, on the other hand, was saddled with a laundry list of demands stretching far beyond mere fat modification. (And to sweeten the deal while also boosting compliance, the group was showered with foodie freebies.) As outlined in the trial's 1966 publication, the experimental diet was made up of the following:[34]

- Sardines canned in cod liver oil—supplied for free

- Soybean oil, supplied free on request, to cook with or to take as "medicine"—whichever was needed to reach half a liter per week

- An advisory to restrict meat as much as possible—and if consumed, to trim it of any visible fat. (As a replacement, the participants could eat "whale beef" and poultry)

- Fish of all types, including shellfish

- Skim milk only. Whole milk and cream were to be completely eliminated. Exceptions were allowed for lightening coffee and for a single one-deciliter serving of milk with Sunday dessert

- Lowfat cheese in place of full-fat cheese

- One egg with yolk, allowed once a week. Egg whites could be used in cooking

- Common types of bread, including wheat and rye, as long as they didn't contain whole milk or "extra margarine"

- Brown sugar in place of "pure" sugar

- All "foods of vegetable origin," such as salads, beans, peas, cabbage, carrots, fruit, and nuts—but no coconut

- Butter and margarine substitutes made from a mixture of skim milk powder, soybean oil, salt, and food coloring. (Lard, shortening, and olive oil were also discouraged)

- Alcoholic and non-alcoholic beverages in moderation

- A daily multiple vitamin free of cost. Each tablet contained 5000 IU of vitamin A, 500 IU of vitamin D, 2 mg thiamine, 3 mg riboflavin, 20 mg niacin, 2mg pyridoxine, and 3mg calcium pantoteneate]

Let's stand back for a moment and join hands for a critical thinking pow-wow and consider all the changes made to the control group's diet.

The Oslo Diet-Heart Study increased:
- Intake of fish and shellfish
- Omega-3 intake—up to extra 5 grams per day[35]
- Intake of salads, beans, peas, cabbage, carrots, fruit, and nuts
- Intake of fat-soluble vitamins A and D from the cod liver oil in sardine packs (as well as calcium from the sardines' bones)
- Emphasized brown bread over white

The Oslo Diet-Heart Study decreased or eliminated:
- Decreased sugar consumption
- Decreased trans fat intake by 7 grams per day[36]
- Eliminated whole milk and cream

How the Oslo Diet-Heart Study represents itself:
- As a study that proves that replacing saturated fat with vegetable oils will make you healthier.

Do you see the problem here?

Actually, the Oslo Diet-Heart Study was a pretty decent trial. Unfortunately, *it's not a trial that tested the diet-heart hypothesis.* Trying to cite it as such doesn't change that fact any more than claiming Elvis plays Texas Hold 'Em with you on Sundays makes him not dead. It just isn't true.

Nonetheless, the study stands as a "landmark study"—towering alongside the Finnish Mental Hospital Trial—that supposedly bolsters the high PUFA, low-saturated-fat dietary recommendations (still pushed by the USDA and other health authorities today), while ignoring the other dietary variables included in the study.

Let's now examine the study's follow-up. After a five-year jaunt in the trial, the diets of the participants were no longer under the careful watch of researchers. Instead, the men were given some dietary tips to take to heart, and that's it.

Those who had been in the high PUFA experimental group were advised to stick with the cholesterol-lowering diet they'd mastered during the previous years. And those who had been in the control group were told they might benefit from trimming some fat from their diet, but weren't given a lick of guidance beyond that.

So essentially, all the men in the study were released back into the dietary wilderness and allowed to roam free, choosing to stick with the study's diet—or not. By the time the eleven-year follow-up rolled around six years later, heart disease mortality remained significantly different between the two groups. Yet the difference in *total* mortality between them was less impressive—failing to meet any statistical significance ($p = 0.35$).

Without knowing how the men ate during those six post-study years (and whether the former PUFA group stuck with their learned menu or abandoned it), it's impossible to draw any conclusions about the impact of the Oslo study on longer-term mortality. But the results of the follow-up raise questions about what the overall mortality trends were for those five years of intensive dietary changes—figures sadly unreported by Leren.

As we'll see in a few other studies outlined in this chapter, rates of cancer mortality would become particularly valuable to examine.

Los Angeles Veterans Administration Study

The Oslo study wasn't the last problematic diet-heart-testing creature in line, either. In 1969, the results of *another* study—this one spanning eight years and, like the Finnish Mental Hospital Trial, swapping saturated-fat-rich foods for polyunsaturated oils—were published in *Circulation*. And it sang a much more alarming tune.

Commonly known as the LA Veterans Administration Study, the trial studied 846 elderly men living in a veteran's home where their food intake could be rigorously monitored (and, due to their age, the men were unlikely to pack their bags and vamoose mid-study).

While the control group received a standard American diet consisting of 40 percent fat with only a tenth of that fat being polyunsaturated, the experimental group quadrupled their PUFA intake at the expense of saturated fat.

Both groups maintained roughly the same total fat intake, only the experimental group cut their dietary cholesterol by nearly half. The diet breakdowns shaped up as follows on the next page.

Calories per day
Control group: 2496
Experimental group: 2496

Protein (grams per day)
Control group: 96.3
Experimental group: 97.4

Fat (percent of total calories)
Control group: 40.1
Experimental group: 38.9

Cholesterol (mg per day)
Control group: 653
Experimental group: 365

Polyunsaturated fat (percent of total fatty acids)
Control group: 10 (or 4 percent of total calories)
Experimental group: 39.5 (or a bit over 15 percent of total calories)

In addition to successfully controlling diet variables, the study had a number of other strengths.

Randomized? Check. The men were ushered into the experimental group or control group via randomization.

Double blind? Check. Neither the men nor the doctors evaluating their causes of death knew who received which diet.

But the study's main weakness was that, despite the randomization process doing a stellar job of keeping baseline characteristics evenly matched between the control and experimental groups, a dispropor-tionate number of smokers ended up in the control group compared to the experimental. Keep this in mind as we trek through the next few paragraphs, because—if anything—it predisposed the control group to less favorable health outcomes.

The first several years looked mighty promising for the high PUFA veterans—predictable, one supposes,

FACTOID: Eighteen percent of deaths in the experimental group were from cancer, compared to a bit fewer than 10 percent in the control group. Just to flex our stats muscles, that's an *absolute* change of 8 percent, but a *relative* change of 80 percent.

if you follow food-pyramid wisdom. The cholesterol levels of the experimental group dropped by almost 13 percent—a reduction that held steady for the full eight years of the trial and would've knocked the socks off any cholesterol-leery doctor.

Likewise, the experimental group's heart disease mortality sank relative to the control group's. Had the control and experimental groups been locked in a literal race, the experimental group might be the hare: speeding out of sight from the tortoise and declaring a premature victory. But behind the scenes, something formidable was happening.

Despite the experimental group's advantage on the heart disease front, their overall mortality was pretty evenly matched with the control group. That's because despite dying less from heart disease, the high PUFA group was dying *more* from something else.

And it just so happened to be cancer.

By the seventh year of the study, the high PUFA group's cancer mortality took a sharp upward turn. In the eighth year, those deaths rose even more, with similarly striking speed. And in the ninth year? Oops, we don't know—because that's when the researchers, unaware of the surprising turn of events, ended the study.

Although the researchers didn't realize what was going on until it was too late—losing the opportunity to see if cancer continued to rise in the group that was supposed to be healthiest had they extended the trial—they *did* realize the issue was too significant to ignore.

FACTOID: Today, food manufacturers can still slap a "zero trans fat" label on their foods even if it contains up to half a gram per serving. While that might not seem like a lot, it can add up quickly in products like cooking sprays, whose serving size is even *less* than half a gram—making it legally possible for the product to consist of nothing but trans fat and still be marketed as free of it.

And thus was born another paper titled "Incidence of Cancer in Men on a Diet High in Polyunsaturated Fat," published in *The Lancet* in 1971.[37] In it, two of the study's researchers, Morton Lee Pearce and Seymour Dayton, shift their focus away from the PUFA diet's reduction in heart disease mortality and onto the disturbing excess of lives it claimed from cancer.

In describing the phenomenon, the researchers confessed their own

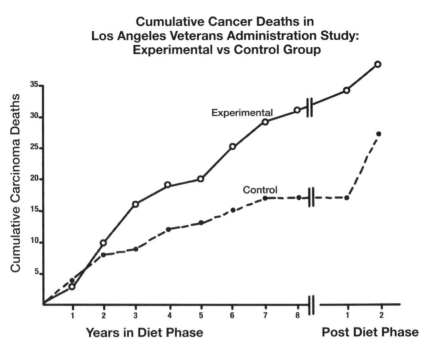

**Cumulative Cancer Deaths in
Los Angeles Veterans Administration Study:
Experimental vs Control Group**

TABLE 6. Data from Morton Lee Pearce and Seymour Dayton, "Incidence of Cancer in Men on a Diet High in Polyunsaturated Fat," *The Lancet* (1971). After two years on a high-PUFA diet, the experimental group saw an unexpected spike in cancer deaths that lasted throughout the study.

surprise about what happened. "We anticipated that [the experimental group's] deaths would be due to a variety of competing causes in these elderly men," they explained in their paper. But the non-cardiac deaths weren't evenly dispersed among those various causes. They wrote:

> Subsequently we reviewed all our data with regard to deaths from causes other than atherosclerotic complications, especially when we read of experiments which association unsaturated-fat feeding with an increased incidence of spontaneous and induced neoplasms in animals.... We found a higher than expected incidence of carcinoma deaths in the experimental group.

With a *p-value* of 0.06, that finding was just on the cusp of statistical significance—not powerful enough to shout from the rooftops with conviction, but clearly pointing toward something important. And if the trial's mortality patterns had continued moving in the direction they veered during the last few years of the experiment, the difference in cancer death rate may well have become even more compelling.

The cancer-based offshoot paper, though, added a new chunk of data as well: the two-year follow-up experience of returning the study's surviving participants to their institution's standard diet. The results here, too, were intriguing. For the first year after the trial ended and everyone resumed a fairly similar diet, the men who'd spent eight years on the high PUFA menu *still* saw a disproportionate rate of cancer mortality—four deaths compared to zero among men who'd been in the control group. But by the next year, that trend was gone, and the former-experimental-group's cancer rate had dropped below that of the control group. The clustering of cancer deaths following high PUFA intake, with a carryover effect for about a year, was undeniable.

The researchers scoured their brains—and their data—in search of an explanation. But nary another factor could account for the rise in cancers clearly associated with the high PUFA group. Having exhausted all avenues possible with the information they'd collected, the researchers somberly concluded: "There is no apparent non-dietary explanation for the higher frequency of carcinoma deaths in the experimental group."

One conundrum, which clearly left the researchers befuddled, was the fact that these findings seemed to contradict other data available at the time. The handful of similar studies that'd been completed by the early seventies failed to find increases in cancer deaths among high PUFA experimental groups.

Yet as the researchers explained, none of those studies had lasted as long as the LA Veteran Administrations trial. (And indeed, it wasn't until the tail end of the study that the cancer trends became most alarming.)

Also, several of the seemingly disparate trials—for example, the Oslo Diet-Heart Study—were confounded by other dietary changes, another hadn't published cancer data yet, and virtually all of the studies differed in terms of design and the type of folks under examination.

In the end, the study raised more questions than it brought answers. Would the PUFA-cancer connection keep gaining strength

THE IRONY OF TYRANNY

In 1984, The Center for Science in the Public Interest (CSPI)—an activist group known for its aggressive "food cop" tactics—made a royal blunder. With the anti-saturated-fat movement in full swing, the CSPI pressured the fast-food industry into replacing traditional, saturated frying oils with "healthier" oils rich in trans fats. The effort was a success: coconut oil, palm oil, and beef tallow promptly vanished from fast-food chains across the nation, while partially hydrogenated oils took their place. But in 1993, the CSPI was back in the complaint line—this time to reverse its own damage. Accepting no part of the blame, the CSPI filed a lawsuit against KFC for using those very trans-fat rich oils they'd pressured the chain into using—which now had firm evidence of being hazardous.[47]

if the trial had lasted longer than eight years? What would happen if those participants had stuck with their high PUFA diets for one more year? Five years? Ten?

Unfortunately, we don't know for sure—because there hasn't been a single controlled study lasting long enough to find out. The only ongoing experiment, it seems, is the American public—and other Westernized populations with similar food trends—as we're federally coaxed toward diets higher in PUFAs than the human body has ever experienced ever before in history.

Fat or Fiction?

Having been thoroughly alerted to the potentially nefarious role of PUFA's, the AHA released a science advisory in 2009 titled "Omega-6 Fatty Acids and Risk of Cardiovascular Disease." It acknowledged other individuals and groups that recommended that people should reduce their omega-6 PUFA intake. The purpose of this advisory, the AHA stated, was "to review evidence on the relationship between omega-6 PUFAs and the risk of CHD and cardiovascular disease."

Their conclusion was unequivocal. According to the AHA paper, the collective data from both human and animal studies shows that consuming 5 to 10 percent of total energy in the form of omega-6 PUFAs is not only healthy, but that "higher intakes appear to be safe and may be even more beneficial." (Continued on page 178.)

A FATTY ACID BALANCING ACT

Although there's no standard recommendation for total omega-6 or omega-3 intake, the ideal ratio for these fats is generally thought to be around 1 to 1—that is, an equal intake of both. That's approximately the ratio we encountered during the Paleolithic era, and the ratio most hunter-gatherer groups still consume today. (An excellent discussion of this can be found in Artemis P. Simopoulos's paper "Omega-6/Omega-3 Essential Fatty Acid Ratio and Chronic Diseases," published in *Food Reviews International* in 2004.)

Alas, polyunsaturated fats—omega-3 and omega-6 included—are rather fragile creatures: their molecular structure, full of double bonds that earn them their "poly" (*many*) label, makes them more prone to oxidation than other types of fat. And for you, that means it's far wiser to keep total PUFA intake low by *reducing* your omega-6 intake to match omega-3, rather than raising omega-3 intake to astronomical heights to compensate for a diet rich in omega-6.

But for the sake of comparison, let's paint a real-world picture of just how tough it'd be to get a 1 to 1 ratio of these fats if you're still eating industrial vegetable oils. How many ounces of salmon—perhaps our most famous omega-3 rich food—would you need to balance out one ounce (two tablespoons) of the following common oils? (You'd easily hit that one-ounce quota with a single serving of salad dressing.)

(Numbers are based on 1 ounce of cooked, wild Atlantic salmon—which has an omega-3 content of 724 mg per serving and an omega-6 content of 62 mg per serving. The amount of *farmed* salmon you'd need to eat would be even higher, since their corn-and-soy-rich diets give their bodies a lower omega-3 content than their wild counterparts.)

Soybean oil: 19 ounces of salmon

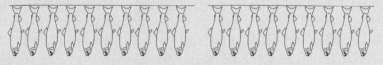

Corn oil: 22 ounces of salmon

Cottonseed oil: 22 ounces of salmon

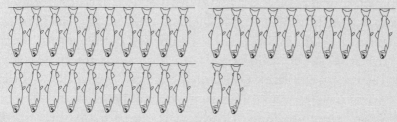

Safflower oil: 32 ounces of salmon

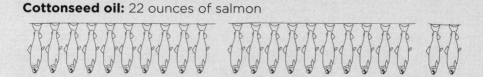

Sunflower oil: 12 ounces of salmon

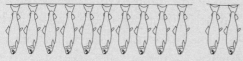

Peanut oil: 13 ounces of salmon

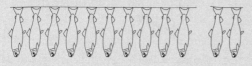

Sesame oil: 17 ounces of salmon

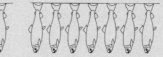

Butter: 1 ounce of salmon

TABLE 7. Information sourced from NutritionData.self.com.

In conclusion, they warned that reducing omega-6 PUFA intakes from what Americans already consume "would be more likely to increase than to decrease risk for CHD."

Although the AHA tends to project an aura of cool objectivity, and their declaration of omega-6 safety might seem like the final word on the matter, there are a few reasons to question the paper's validity. For starters, it's worth taking a closer look at just who penned that report.

As noted in the paper's "Disclosures" section, the lead author— William Harris—received significant funding from the bioengineering giant Monsanto, in addition to serving as a consultant for them. In fact, Harris had been hoisted aboard Monsanto's research ship to study the company's latest creation: an omega-3 enhanced soybean modified with genes from primrose flowers and bread mold.[38]

Shortly before the AHA released their omega-6 advisory, Harris published a study in *Lipids* showing that Monsanto's engineered soybeans could boost omega-3 levels in the blood—while also supplying the ample omega-6 content.[39] (Since then, Harris has authored additional papers supporting the benefits of Monsanto's new soybean oil as a promising land-based alternative to marine oils.[40,41])

Likewise, two additional authors of the AHA paper—plus all three of its reviewers—had received grants, been given other financial support, or served on advisory boards for places with a vested interest in PUFAs being healthful. Four of the authors and reviewers, in fact, had connections to Unilever—the maker of *I Can't Believe It's Not Butter* and other margarines that serve as some of the highest sources of omega-6 fats in the Western world.

Of course, financial connections don't automatically mean information is unreliable or biased beyond repair. Researchers have to get funding from *somewhere,* and often it's corporations and other profitable entities willing to dish out that dough. Yet it's hard to deny that producers of high-omega-6 foods would benefit from a major-league player like the American Heart Association endorsing—even indirectly—their products. And in the context of existing PUFA literature, the AHA's kindness toward omega-6 fats does seem suspect.

Luckily, it was an oddity not lost on other scientists. After the AHA released their advisory, researchers from around the globe emerged to contest its conclusions. One commentary in the *British Journal of Nutrition* asked rhetorically whether the advisory was "evidence based or biased evidence," pointing out that the AHA drew many of its omega-6 conclusions from studies that suffered major design flaws, were confounded by changes in omega-3 consumption, or otherwise failed to support the healthfulness of a high omega-6 intake specifically.[42] The UK, in fact, had been warning for years that "there is reason to be cautious about high intakes of n-6 PUFAs," going on to say that those whose diets already contain 10 percent or more of this fat shouldn't play with fire by increasing it further.[43]

Other criticisms of the AHA's omega-6 cheerleading abounded. Artemis Simopoulos—President of the Center for Genetics, Nutrition, and Health—also contested the AHA's advisory, noting that the levels of omega-6 PUFAs currently in the American diet ought to be *reduced*, not held steady or raised. Explaining that humans had never in our existence experienced a diet high in omega-6 fats until the last fifty years or so, she called the modern omega-6 frenzy "an artificial way and a general experiment, being done without any scientific evidence."[44]

In all, the AHA advisory cites a select few papers to support a positive view of PUFAs, while dismissing a larger body of work calling the safety of skyrocketing intakes into question. The advisory states: "In human studies, higher plasma levels of omega-6 PUFAs, mainly AA, were associated with decreased plasma levels of serum proinflammatory markers, particularly interleukin-6 and interleukin-1 receptor antagonist, and increased levels of anti-inflammatory markers, particularly transforming growth factor-β."

In simple English, the advisory is basically saying that in the human studies they reviewed they found that the more omega-6 fatty acids in the blood, the fewer inflammatory markers in the body. To back up this statement, the advisory cites a single observational study from Northern Italy, in which the population—residents of the Rifredi district in Florence—had an average PUFA intake of only 2.9 percent of total energy.[45] Considering that the US consumes closer to 7 percent, the Italian study is a stretch as evidence for the safety (much less *benefit)* of PUFA oils in a nation that consumes more than twice the amount. What's more, the Italian study was conducted in a region where 99.6 percent of the population reported a staggeringly low total PUFA intake.[46] Given all of that, why is the advice to consume plenty of vegetable oils—especially those rich in omega-6—still blasting in our ears?

The reason is twofold.

First, from a health standpoint, PUFAs allure come from their cholesterol-lowering effect. They make lipid profiles look better on paper (at least in theory) and offer a sense of security matched only by statins. After all, *lower your cholesterol to save your heart* has become Western medicine's oft-recited battle cry.

And second, vegetable oil is financially appealing. Since its very inception with Procter and Gamble back in 1912, polyunsaturated plant fats have indeed been unabashedly promoted as "healthy for the wallet" long before any "healthy for the body" arguments entered the scene. As unfortunate as it sounds, the budget-saving aspect may be PUFAs' greatest appeal.

The Problem With Modern PUFA Studies

If increased oxidation caused by PUFAs really is as problematic as some argue, its effect may not be linear. For the sake of illustration, let's imagine running a fairly villainous experiment where you give one person a bottle of cyanide to drink, and you give another person two bottles to drink. Even though Person B drank a doubled dose of poison, Person B won't be any *more* dead than Person A, who drank a single dose. And Person B won't be dead any faster—because both A and B still drank enough poison to elicit the maximum effect.

Likewise, in a realm industrialized vegetable oils, there comes a point where cell membranes simply cannot become any more saturated with PUFAs, no matter how many gallons of corn oil consumed. Increasing intake past the threshold—which is, quite possibly, a level the typical American diet has already met or exceeded—won't do significantly more harm, because the damage is already maxed out.

For this reason, observational studies of Western nations are one of the worst ways to seek answers about PUFA consumption. Thanks to the nearly ubiquitous presence of high-omega-6 oils in our diet, even the lowest-PUFA eaters of the bunch may be consuming levels above that damage-causing threshold. The most compelling PUFA-related health changes won't come until we can get our diets back down to normal levels, down to where they were at the turn of the twentieth century, before Procter met Gamble.

10
Meet
Your Meat

FOR THE SAKE OF FULL DISCLOSURE: I'm not a big meat eater. I personally eat land-roaming animals about once a month, at roughly the same pace of full moons and freshly announced celebrity pregnancies (not that correlation equals causation). In my case, the reason is a simple combination of taste preferences, the results of ongoing self-guinea-pigging, and a decade of vegetarianism that left my meat-cooking skills on par with that of a seven year old. My meat forays are usually a matter of social situations or inexplicable steak cravings that arise after watching the Food Network.

That said, I'm not here to tilt you one way or another on the meat fence with anecdotes from my own life. Meat is obviously a controversial food ensnared in various health, environmental, ethical, and even religious issues; the goal of this book isn't to moralize about its consumption or pass along my own preferences as gospel. Instead, we should let the science speak for itself. This chapter will focus on presenting the most objective view possible—free from wishful thinking, free from preexisting ethical stances, free from the influence of prevailing but unsubstantiated belief—on a food so often under fire (or over it, if your Weber grill is involved).

So enough about me. Let's talk about meat.

What's the Matter with Meat?
Ever since McGovern's *Dietary Goals* of 1977, the message to eat less red meat has been ringing loud and clear in American ears. And even if the nation weren't pulled under the spell of public policy, science itself certainly seems to cast this brand of protein in a shady light. Observational research manages to pump out an endless ream of warnings that meat consumption—particularly of the red or processed variety—is

associated with higher rates of overall mortality, cancer, heart disease, and other chronic diseases.

Although it can be awfully tempting to cite the limitations of observational studies and shove that research under the "correlation doesn't imply causation" banner, there actually may be some valid pathways connecting meat with some of the health problems it seems to associate with—at least in certain contexts. Let's take a gander at what those could be.

Muscle Meat Mania

Stroll through your local grocery store, and the meat aisle will probably follow a classic pattern. *Sirloin. Short loin. Rib, Flank. Chuck. Round. Brisket.* In other words, a raw, packaged wonderland of *muscle meat*—the cuts that, for one reason or another, have become our favored forms of animal flesh. Anything outside of the muscle-meat umbrella tends to be relegated to a smaller refrigerated pocket rarely graced by our shopping carts.

But it hasn't always been that way. A peek into recipes from the days of yore—such as the Crisco cookbook we touched on earlier—reveals an assortment of animal ingredients we might find gag-worthy today: brains, eyes, kidneys, thymus gland, pancreas, tails, tendons, hooves, bones, and other grizzly bits many of us would hardly consider edible. Yet in contrast to our current aversion to these foods, they once enjoyed eons as the most cherished part of a kill. Even today, faced with a fresh carcass, hunter-gatherer groups and other non-industrialized communities—not to mention virtually every meat-eating animal under the sun—make beelines for organs and bones, sometimes even discarding the very tenderloin you might dish out $12.99 a pound for. An analysis of traditional diet and food preferences among the Australian Aborigines, for instance, showed that virtually every part of the animal was eaten, including "the small fat depots and organ meats (which were highly prized), bone marrow, some stomach contents, peritoneal fluid, and blood."[1] How often do those delicacies land on your own plate?

There's a big problem with our current muscle-meat-crazed state of affairs. A few of them, actually:

Amino acid showdown. Muscle meat is notoriously high in the amino acid *methionine* (pronounced meh-THY-uh-neen), whereas the oft-neglected parts of an animal—most notably skin, bones, tendons, and connective tissue—are rich in the amino acid *glycine*. Although methionine isn't an inherent dietary villain, it can stir up trouble if it's not balanced out by a proper array of other nutrients. For one, a high methionine intake increases your need for vitamin B12, vitamin B6, folate, choline, and betaine, which help neutralize *homocysteine*, one of methionine's most noxious byproducts (with a much-debated link to vascular disease, to boot).[2] So if your meat-eating habits skew too far towards the muscle side, you might need to up your intake of certain nutrients to compensate.

What's more, methionine can drain your body's glycine stores—so if you're eating a diet heavy in muscle meats without chowing down on the rest of the animal (or eating a whole lot of Jell-O), your methionine to glycine ratio will be tragically off kilter. Only by eating "nose to tail"—that includes the animal's bones and skin and organs and cartilage—can you achieve an amino acid ratio optimal for human health. (Intriguingly, in animal models methionine restriction has the same life-extending properties as calorie restriction. In some breeds of rats, identical perks emerge from supplementing a high-methionine diet with glycine.[3] More human study would be needed before determining if our own species might also benefit from glycine supplementation, too.)

Nutritional robbery. A quick comparison between 100 grams of muscle meat and equal weight of brain, heart, liver, kidney, or other organs shows that muscle is a sad lightweight as far as vitamins and minerals go. While it may be rich in protein and iron, muscle tissue misses out on a host of other goodies like copper, vitamin A, potassium, magnesium, pantothenic acid, and more. Organs are some of the most nutritionally dense foods in existence—and skipping them for chicken breast or ground beef is a lost opportunity for first-class nourishment.

Regardless of whether some components of meat are legitimately harmful, there's little doubt that America is doing meat *wrong*. Ditto for nearly every other nation affluent enough for prime cuts of muscle to dominate the animal-food scene. By favoring muscle meats over the traditional "nose to tail" way of eating, we're losing out on one of nature's most nutrient-dense resources. The solution? Don't stop at the T-bone steak: make an effort to brew glycine-rich broth from bones, venture into the culinary world of organ meats like liver and heart, cook with skin and tendons and connective tissue, and expand your view of which parts of the animal get invited to dinner.

Modern Cooking Methods

As we've explored in our sagas of Ancel Keys, Framingham, and the formation of the 1977 *Dietary Goals,* the two biggest strikes against meat—its saturated fat and cholesterol content—aren't necessarily the agents of doom we've been led to believe. But that doesn't mean meat is off the hook for good. In fact, we have a mounting pile of evidence at our fingertips showing that the *way* we treat our meat, particularly in the kitchen, may be responsible for some of those suspicious links between meat and disease popping up in observational studies.

Picture this. You pick out a thick, good-looking sirloin steak at the butcher, bring it home, fire up the barby, and throw your newly acquired meat over an open flame, constrained only by the scorching hot slats of a grill. (Feel free to baste it in something delicious in the process.) There it remains until all the meaty bits mar into a new assortment of compounds. Congratulations! It's well done. And potentially carcinogenic, to boot.

Indeed, every time you cook meat at very high temperatures, especially exposed to direct flame, you invite carcinogenic properties into your meal. Some of the compounds generated by harsh cooking include:

1. Heterocyclic amines (HAs). These gnarly compounds form when amino acids, sugars, and creatine—a chemical in meat—react at high temperatures. Typically, it takes cooking meat above 300 degrees, or to the point of well-doneness, for HAs to become an issue.[4]

2. Polycyclic aromatic hydrocarbons (PAHs). PAHs form during grilling, when meat juices and fat drip into the fire below, causing PAH-containing flames to leap up and coat the surface of the meat. You can find PAHs in nearly any food that's been charred or smoked.

Despite making food pretty delicious, HAs and PAHs can result in DNA mutations after being "bioactivated" by certain enzymes in your body—creating a setting ripe for cancer formation. In animal studies, supplementing critters' diets with HAs results in cancer on a fairly consistent basis—particularly colon cancer, skin cancer, breast cancer, and prostate cancer.[5,6,7,8] Leukemia and lung cancer, too, have cropped up in rodents after high exposure to PAHs.[9] We've already hashed out why rodent studies can be misleading, of course—but since we can't ethically force humans to eat substances suspected of causing cancer, long-term controlled trials in our own species are nil.

A Kinder, Gentler Heat
The image of blackening meat over fire might seem like one of those ancient, primitive practices. But in reality, early humans often employed much gentler cooking methods. One method was "stone boiling," which involved placing stones next to a fire source until they were toasty hot, and then dumping them into a water vessel to get it boiling. Other methods included cooked leaf-wrapped meat over hot rocks and boiling food in hide-lined pits.[20]

That said, the jury's still out about how well those animal studies transfer to humans. For one, it's excruciatingly difficult to measure HA and PAH exposure in our diets with much accuracy, especially from food frequency questionnaires.[10] Second, the enzymes that metabolize HAs and PAHs have different activity levels in different people, so a level of HA intake that's harmful for one person might be benign to the next. And third, folks face environmental exposure to HAs and PAHs from sources beyond food—in rain water, cigarette smoke, diesel exhaust, and airborne particles. So even if we could gauge dietary intake with dazzling precision, there's no telling what the net exposure would be when factoring in all the other places HAs and PAHs may lurk.[11] Collectively, that all makes it pretty hard to get clear data on the subject.

Nonetheless, observational studies on humans *do* tend to show sturdy links between well-done, barbecued, or fried meat and certain cancers—particularly pancreatic, colorectal, and prostate.[12,13,14] In fact, the "meat will kill you" studies that manage to differentiate between various cooking methods generally show that high-temperature-cooked meat is largely driving the disease associations.

So what's an omnivore to do? Here are a few tips:

- Use gentle cooking methods like stewing and steaming for the bulk of your meat.
- Limit charred or smoked foods, meat or otherwise—and cut off charred portions before consumption.
- Avoid directly exposing meat to open fire or temperatures above 300 degrees.
- Use marinades including lemon juice, onions, and garlic, or red wine—which can cut HA content dramatically.[15,16,17]
- If you're going to grill or barbecue, partially cook food using gentler methods before putting it on the grill.
- When cooking on a high-heat surface, continuously turn meat over to avoid buildup of HAs and PAHs—don't let it sit stagnant with only occasional flipping.

Iron Overload

Another potential suspect in observational meat-and-disease links is none other than *iron.* Popeye might've convinced the school-age crowd that spinach rules, but for most of us, red meat holds the iron throne. And often, we think of that as a good thing: iron carries with it the image of vigor and strength, and it seems quite sensible to stuff ourselves with it.

But when it comes to iron, more isn't always better. In America, about 10 percent of the population—or one out of every ten people—is affected by *hereditary hemochromatosis,* a disorder that causes your body to absorb too much iron from the food you eat and store it in your organs. Men of Northern European—especially Celtic—descent are at the highest risk. Over time, the excess iron builds up in your joints, liver, heart, pancreas, and other organs, ultimately raising your risk of getting cancer, liver cirrhosis, diabetes, osteoporosis, heart problems, and other conditions.[18] (Due to the time it takes for iron to accumulate to toxic levels, symptoms of hemochromatosis often don't crop up until midlife—and in the early stages include easy-to-misdiagnose signs like weakness, lethargy, joint pain, and abdominal pain.)

While the iron in meat is fairly innocuous for folks without the condition, those whose bodies *are* stuck in iron-absorption overdrive should take some precautions. Cutting down on iron-rich foods like red meat, of course, is one option—though you can also curb iron absorption by pairing high-iron meals with a cup of coffee or tea, which reduce iron absorption by 35 percent and 62 percent, respectively.[19] Another route is simply donating blood—which is the usual prescription for folks who've built up iron stores to unhealthy levels.

While it's become fashionable in some alternative health circles—especially those taking pride in rebelling against the USDA's anti-saturated fat advice—to go hog-wild on bacon and steak, doing so unscrupulously might not be a great idea. Even with the weaknesses associated with the observational research driving our major meat-and-disease associations, we *have* identified some legitimate pathways through which meat could pose harm. Luckily, it's not too hard to dodge those problems with a little planning. To follow are a few ways to balance your muscle meat intake.

- Include animal organs and other offal in your diet

- Make use of glycine-rich foods like bone broth and cartilage

- Cook meat gently instead of clobbering it with high heat and open flame

- And finally, if you suffer from an iron storage disorder like hemochromatosis, be cautious with high-iron foods in your diet—or learn to love bloodletting. Since hemochromatosis tends to be "silent" up until midlife (at which point its more nefarious symptoms can crop up), the only way to know if you have it is by getting one of two blood tests: serum transferrin saturation and serum ferritin. The results of those tests will show whether you have iron overload and help your doctor make a diagnosis.

11
Herbivore's Dilemma

In September of 2010, Bill Clinton—a slimmer, whiter-haired version of his former presidential self—sat down for an interview on CNN and divulged a story near to his heart, quite literally. After a quadruple bypass interrupted his book tour six years earlier, Clinton had found himself under the knife yet again: this time for two stents to prop open a vein that had already re-filled with plaque.

Once a proud connoisseur of chicken enchiladas and lemon chess pie, Clinton's second hospital jaunt was enough to turn him onto a greener, leaner, more fibrous path. "I went on essentially a plant-based diet," Clinton told CNN's Wolf Blitzer. The former commander in chief described his new menu as an array of beans, legumes, vegetables, and fruits, with a plant-based protein supplement each morning thrown in for good measure. Recounting the research that inspired him to abandon his meat-loving ways, Clinton remarked:

> So I did all this research and I saw that 82 percent of the people since 1986 who have gone on a plant-based diet—no dairy, no meat of any kind, chicken, turkey … 82 percent of the people who have done that have begun to heal themselves. Their arterial blockage cleans up; the calcium deposit around their heart breaks up.[1]

The impressive "82 percent" he cited—albeit out of context—came from Dean Ornish's Lifestyle Heart Trial, the first study to show heart disease could actually be *reversed* without the use of drugs or surgery. Of course, the trial was also famously *multifactorial*—ushering participants through a slew of lifestyle changes ranging from stress reduction to exercise to smoking cessation. But just as we saw with the Pritikin program in the 1970s, it was the study's near-vegan dietary component that cemented into public awareness.

Clinton was just one of a growing number of Americans nixing the USDA food pyramid's already-spurned meat and dairy tier and replacing it with more vegetables, fruits, grains, and legumes. Indeed, one of the hottest contenders for the nation's next dietary direction is the *plant-based diet* movement, which posits that better health will come from shifting the country's menu even further plantward than federal guidelines have steered us.

The umbrella of plant-based eating encompasses everything from vegetarianism to veganism to more flexible whole-foods diets that simply keep meat, egg, and dairy intake as low as possible—options all united by the belief that plants are the best fuel for the human body. Of course, many people adopt vegetarian and vegan lifestyles for reasons other than health, including ethical considerations, religious or spiritual mandates, and environmental concerns. For our purposes here, I'll speak chiefly from the nutritional perspective.

So apart from their snowballing popularity, are plant-based diets our best bet for helping the human body not just survive, but thrive? To answer this question, we need to pop back in time to look at how plant-based menus earned their "healthy diet" stripes in the first place. It's not as straightforward a journey as you might think.

A Journey of Comas, Visions, and Cereal

While vegetarianism has ancient global roots and a hard-to-pinpoint beginning on planet earth, we owe its birth in America largely to the Seventh-day Adventists, a twenty-four-million-member religion famous for its endorsement of healthful living and vegetarian eating. The church traces its roots back to the Millerite movement of the early nineteenth century—an American Christian sect that promised Christ would return on October 22, 1844, and left thousands of believers "sick with disappointment" when he was a no-show. After their savior's failed return, which became aptly known as the Great Disappointment, a number of Millerites disbanded and faded into oblivion. But the loyal remainders recouped their loss by claiming the whole ordeal had stemmed from a scriptural misinterpretation. That group of believers would later become known as the Seventh-day Adventists.

Yet the Adventists' health and diet message didn't take shape until nearly two decades later, largely to the credit of one woman: Ellen

Gould White. At the age of nine, White—a twin from a devout Millerite family—had been clobbered in the face by a stone from a rowdy classmate, knocking her into a three-week coma. Although the incident cut short her schooling and left her permanently disfigured, White eventually accepted her experience as the "the cruel blow which blighted the joys of earth" and turned her eyes toward heaven.[2]

Some critics suggest the accident left her with a traumatic brain injury and catalepsy, leading to seizures and hallucinations she would later interpret as divine prophecies.[3] But White herself believed the experience was a fated step in the unfolding of her spirituality. Amid the bolt-from-the-blue visions that speckled her entire adult life, she claimed to channel health guidelines of divine origin—including not only edicts for adequate sleep, sunshine, rest, and social connection, but also for vegetarian eating and adherence to the Biblical dietary laws prescribed in Leviticus.

White's first major vision about health gripped her on June 6, 1863—a moment she described as a "great light from the Lord," in which she saw God's people urged to abstain from all forms of flesh food.[4] And as the years and visions rolled on, White increasingly saw meat as a threat to not only physical health, but spiritual health as well. In her 1926 publication "Testimony Studies on Diet and Foods," she described meat as both an agent of disease and a thief of human empathy:

> I have been instructed that flesh food has a tendency to animalize the nature, to rob men and women of that love and sympathy which they should feel for every one, and to give the lower passions control over the higher powers of the being. If meat-eating were ever healthful, it is not safe now. Cancers, tumors, and pulmonary diseases are largely caused by meat-eating.[5]

Likewise, White argued that the "sense of weakness and lack of vitality" people felt upon switching to a vegetarian diet was a *good* thing—proving, essentially, that meat was dangerously stimulating, and any strength it seemed to grant was of a dreadfully unholy nature.[6] The visions were undeniable: meat, White was certain, should not pass through any God-fearing lips.

VEGGIE LABEL JARGON: A TRANSLATOR

Most of us use the word "vegetarian" as shorthand for *lacto-ovo vegetarian*—someone who eats eggs and dairy while eschewing flesh foods. But vegetarians, like ice cream, come in a wide variety of delectable flavors. Here are a few samples:

- Pescetarian. A vegetarian who abstains from all meat but fish.

- Lacto-ovo-pesco-pollo-vegetarian (or any variation therein). "Lacto" means dairy, "ovo" means egg, "pesco" means fish, and "pollo" means chicken. You do the math.

- Vegan. Someone who avoids eating anything of animal origin, including meat, dairy, eggs, and oft-overlooked animal byproducts like gelatin and honey. Many extend their philosophy to other areas of life and abstain from using items containing leather, fur, or feathers, as well as any products tested on animals.

- Raw vegan. Along with steering clear of animal products, raw vegans shun anything that's been cooked or heated above 118 degrees or so—automatically excluding most grains, processed store-bought foods, refined oils, and nearly everything else outside the boundaries of the produce section. (Chief among the health advantages of raw veganism is a reduced risk of stovetop burns.)

- Plant-based diet. To distinguish from the political and lifestyle implications tied with veganism, people eating a vegan (or near-vegan) diet for health reasons often refer to their cuisine as a "plant-based diet." That's the term we'll be using for much of this chapter, too. The phrase whole-food, plant-based diet refers specifically to an eating regimen promoted by some prominent physicians and health advocates as a way to reverse disease.

Although White's prophecies became a cornerstone of the Adventist religion, it was one church member in particular who chiseled her message into the pages of American history. At a time when meat was widely regarded as a pillar for good health and a libido-booster in men, a fellow named John Harvey Kellogg hit the scene with a radically different perspective. Obsessed with physical purity, Kellogg—an Adventist born and raised—argued that, contrary to popular notions of his time, the road to health was paved with vegetables and celibacy. And he spent the majority of his life trying to convince the world of the same.

The inspiration for his mission sprung forth in his youth. At age twelve, during the throes of the Civil War, Kellogg became an apprentice for Ellen White's husband and learned the printing trade—which involved immersing himself in thousands of her vision-extracted words on health and the sanctity of the human body.[7] Inspired by what he learned, Kellogg entered adulthood determined to convert health professionals to his meat-free, sex-free, violence-free ideals.

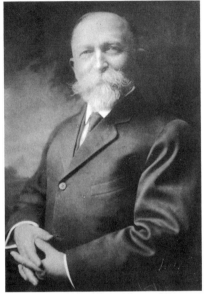

Source: United States Library of Congress

Fig. 13 John Harvey Kellogg, circa 1913, introduced some of the first packaged vegetarian foods, including soy milk and corn flakes.

After earning a medical degree in 1875, Kellogg took over a tiny, Adventist-based medical center and transformed it into the Battle Creek Sanitarium—a spa-slash-health-clinic in Michigan that would eventually house twelve thousand patients at a time, including a celebrity lineup of prominent industrialists, politicians, and other major players in American society. Committed to whipping visitors into tip-top shape, Kellogg invented his own pieces of exercise equipment for the sanitarium's guests to use. And perhaps more famously, he drummed up his own line of vegetarian convenience foods to help nurse visitors back to health—giving to the world, for the first time ever, items like granola, corn flakes, soymilk, and soy-based imitation meats. (His products eventually became property of the Kellogg Company, founded by Kellogg's younger brother, Will Keith Kellogg.)

For decades, Seventh-day Adventism's claim to fame was its transformation of the American breakfast. Meat was still on the menu, but suddenly crunchy cereals were, too, as were expanded options for plant-based foods where the animal kingdom once reigned supreme. Kellogg had failed to win the world over to his celibate, health-obsessed ways, but at least he had a part in filling some bellies with Cornflakes.

But the story doesn't end there. The Adventists officially stole the spotlight not long after Kellogg's passing, when their healthy lifestyles snagged the attention of the scientific community. While Ancel Keys fervently graphed the heart disease rates of various countries, other researchers set their sights on the Adventists, curious why they seemed spared from the chronic diseases plaguing the rest of the country.

Investigators first corralled Adventists into the science world in the 1950s with the launch of the twelve-year Adventist Mortality Study—a project that cranked out our earliest evidence of the Adventists' relative protection against cancer and heart disease.[8] Since then, two other major studies of the Adventist's unique way of life have hit the scene: the Adventist Health Study 1 (AHS-1), which spanned from 1974 to 1988; and the Adventist Health Study 2 (AHS-2), which kicked off in 2002 and is still ongoing. Both offer further confirmation that as a group, the Seventh-day Adventists put the rest of America to shame in nearly every index of health.

One of the reasons the Seventh-day Adventists are such a hot commodity for observational research is that their lifestyles are, at least in theory, fantastically homogenous. Americans at large tend to hop, skip, and yo-yo from diet to diet; drink alcohol excessively or not at all; chain smoke or never smoke; and go to the gym only after pinning their New Year's resolutions to the fridge for a month. That makes for some muddled, confounder-ridden population studies. But by default, the Adventists nearly avoid all those problems. Along with a strong nudge to go vegetarian, the Adventist church teaches its members to abstain from tobacco and alcohol, participate in physical activity, get sunshine and lots of fresh air, and prioritize family life and education (including health education). Adventists are also encouraged to stay away from caffeine, hot condiments, and hot spices. With such guidelines in place—and, for the most part, followed— the biggest area for wiggle room is in how an individual Adventist participates on the no-meat front. Some choose to do the bare minimum and abstain from just pork and shellfish, per the teachings of Jewish law outlined in the book of Leviticus. Others follow a stricter no-animal flesh diet as Ellen White urged.

Indeed, even within the Adventist population, stark differences emerge between folks of different meat-eating persuasions. One analysis found that Adventists following a true vegetarian diet consumed less coffee and doughnuts, and more tomatoes, legumes, nuts, and fruit than the more liberal meat eaters.[9] Likewise, studies of Mormons—who also shun alcohol, tobacco, tea, and coffee, but whose founder never endured any meat-abstinence visions—suggest that they, too, enjoy far-above-average health like the Adventists. Starting in the 1960s and 70s, data emerged showing that Mormons had as little as half the cancer incidence and two-thirds the heart disease mortality of the surrounding population—even when their socioeconomic status, urbanization, and other quality-of-life markers were the same.[10,11] Along with the to-be-expected reduction in cancers linked with smoking, Mormon females had significantly lower rates of breast cancer, cervical cancer, and ovary cancer, while both genders had a one-third reduction in rates of stomach cancer, colon and colorectal cancer, and pancreatic cancer.[12,13]

But what's even more telling is the fact that meat-eating Mormons and vegetarian Adventists tend to live equally as long. When compared to ethnically matched folks outside their religious groups, both Adventist and Mormon men—once their birthday-cake candles start numbering in the thirties—can expect to live about seven years longer than the rest of the population.[14,15]

So what role does meat (or lack thereof) play in the Adventists' longevity? We might never know for sure—but that doesn't stop the media, and even well meaning researchers, from attributing the Adventists' stellar health to their vegetarian ways.

Even among the non-Adventist population, it's a tall order untangling the meatless component of plant-based diets from other entangled variables. Vegetarians, after all, rarely forego meat and call it a day. The decision to drop flesh foods often goes hand-in-hand with a cascade of other nutritional and lifestyle changes known to boost health. In the past couple decades, we've learned that vegetarians tend to exercise more, smoke less, limit alcohol, eat fewer refined grains, eat more vegetables, eat more fruit, eat fewer donuts, and engage in a variety of other behaviors existing independently of meat consumption.[16,17] For vegans, who take vegetarianism one step further by eschewing eggs, dairy, and anything else derived from animals, the increase in positive lifestyle habits is even more dramatic.[18]

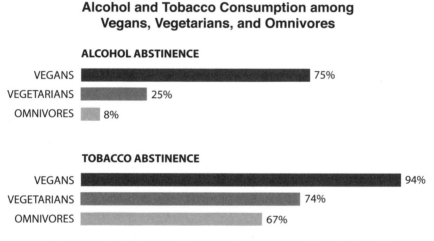

Alcohol and Tobacco Consumption among Vegans, Vegetarians, and Omnivores

ALCOHOL ABSTINENCE

VEGANS	75%
VEGETARIANS	25%
OMNIVORES	8%

TOBACCO ABSTINENCE

VEGANS	94%
VEGETARIANS	74%
OMNIVORES	67%

TABLE 8. Source: Maria Gacek, "Selected Lifestyle and Health Condition Indices of Adults With Varied Models of Eating."

This raises the same question spurred by our studies on Adventists. What is it about vegetarianism that boosts health? Is it the reduction in meat, or the increase in beneficial plant foods? Is it a consequence of diet alone, or do other lifestyle modifications snowball into a giant glob of healthfulness that then tips chronic disease outcomes in a favorable direction? How does vegetarianism work its purported magic?

Unfortunately, we don't yet have clear answers to these questions. The bulk of our vegetarian data comes from population studies— which, if you'll recall, offer descriptive snapshots rather than razor-sharp evidence. It's simply not feasible—mainly for legal and logistical reasons—to conduct the type of widespread, labor-intensive, tightly controlled, and obsessively monitored experiments necessary to gauge how long-term vegetarian lifestyles fare next to identical ones that include meat.

But don't take my word for it. A number of researchers lament this very problem, acknowledging that the benefits of vegetarianism, when they appear, are hard to trace to the exclusion of meat per se. In his 2003 review "The contribution of vegetarian diets to human health," researcher Joan Sabaté—himself a vegetarian—remarked that the benefits of whole plant foods are "possibly more certain than the detrimental effects of meats."[20] Likewise, a 2012 review in *Public Health Nutrition* concluded that going vegetarian isn't the only way to reap the benefits of certain plant foods: simply adding more garden-cultivated superstars to your diet will provide health benefits, regardless of whether you also eschew meat. What's more, no evidence exists to support the idea that simply avoiding meat brings greater health benefits.[21] At least in this case, it's not so much what a diet avoids but what it generously includes. Let's take a closer look.

Do Vegetarians Live Longer?

As we've just learned, vegetarians, when compared to the general population, definitely seem to have a leg up in the longevity race. In fact, at least one vegetarian-dominated population has been crowned a "Blue Zone" because of its famed health and life spans: The Californian city of Loma Linda—home to one of the highest concentrations of Adventists in the US.[22] It shares company with the citizens of Okinawa, Japan, and Sardinia, Italy, as a centenarian hotspot.

For some, this is enough evidence to hop on the veggie wagon. Yet the life-extending advantage of such a lifestyle gets hazy when you begin to draw similar comparisons with health-conscious omnivores. In a prospective study in Germany, researchers spent twenty-one years following almost two thousand vegetarians and their omnivore family members (who were assumed to have been at least partially influenced by the vegetarians' health enthusiasm), only to discover little difference in mortality between the meat eaters and the meat avoiders.[23]

But here's where it gets really interesting: **despite a nonsignificant reduction in deaths from heart disease, the vegetarians actually had slightly *higher* rates of all-cause mortality and cancerous tumors than the omnivores—although both groups in the study fared much better than the German population at large**.

And when the researchers divided the vegetarian group further into lacto-ovo vegetarians and strict vegans, veganism wound up with

THE PLANT-BASED DIET DOCTOR SQUAD: WHO ARE THEY?

John McDougall limits white flour, refined grains, sugar-coated cereals, soft drinks, processed carbohydrates, fruit juice, and vegetable oils.

Neal Barnard forbids vegetable oils, high-glycemic foods, high fructose corn syrup, caloric sweeteners, and fried starches like potato chips and french fries.

Caldwell Esselstyn eschews vegetable oils, refined grains, white flour, and products made from enriched flour such as bread, pasta, bagels, and baked goods; also uses statins to bring patients' cholesterol down below 150 if diet alone doesn't do the trick.

Dean Ornish limits sugar and sugar derivatives, corn syrup, white flour, margarine, vegetable oils, alcohol, and any processed food with more than two grams of fat. His program also includes smoking cessation, peer support, exercise, and stress management through meditation, stretching, and visualization.

Joel Fuhrman limits oil and white potatoes, and strictly rejects sweets, white rice, white flour, and sugar.

the highest mortality risk out of any group in the study. It was a 59 percent higher risk, in fact, than their omnivore brethren. (Given the relatively small number of vegans scooped into the participant pool—only sixty of them total—it's hard to say whether that finding would've held up with a larger sample size, or if it was mostly a matter of random chance.)

Even more intriguing, the study failed to use omnivores that were truly equally matched with their vegetarian counterparts: the meat-eaters reported lower levels of physical activity, greater alcohol consumption, and more than twice the smoking frequency compared to the study participants who ate no meat. Mortality and disease rates, in this case, might be *expected* to turn up in favor of the vegetarian crowd, even though the opposite ended up happening.

And Germany isn't the only seat of such trends. The Health Food Shoppers Study, which followed nearly eleven thousand health-conscious omnivores and vegetarians in the United Kingdom over the course of twenty-four years, found no difference in overall mortality between those who ate meat and those who didn't.[24] Among specific causes of death, the only significant finding was a considerably higher rate of breast cancer mortality among the vegetarians (a death rate ratio of 1.73—or 73 percent greater—in vegetarians compared to meat eaters). That finding had also popped up in an earlier analysis of the cohort, and the study's investigators suggested it could be related to the fact that British vegetarian women were somewhat more likely to stay childfree. A similar study had found that 37 percent of middle-aged female vegetarians had never given birth, compared to only 28 percent of omnivores.[25] Given that childbearing is protective against breast cancer, it's possible vegetarian women's tendency to produce fewer offspring put them at greater risk for the disease.[26] Whether that was enough to explain the higher death rate among vegetarians remains speculation, though.

Similarly, the Oxford Vegetarian Study—which surveyed over eleven thousand vegetarians in the UK, along with their potentially health-savvy friends and relatives—found zero difference in overall mortality between the vegetarians and omnivores over a twenty-year span.[27] As with the Health Food Shoppers Study, only one specific death-cause reached significance: mortality from mental and neurological diseases, which was 146 percent higher among vegetarians than their non-vegetarian kin. (Considering there were only thirty-six deaths from this category in the whole cohort, though, that statistic is probably worth taking with a grain or two of salt; the smaller the sample size, the greater the danger of false or exaggerated trends emerging.)

As a whole, the only vegetarian population with consistently better health outcomes than omnivores comes from the Seventh-day Adventists—an indication that lifestyle factors other than diet are running the show.

What About Veganism?

Could it be that, as a group, vegetarians fail to dazzle the lifespan charts because they're still eating plenty of eggs and dairy? If you've been traipsing through the health world for any length of time, you might have seen that argument before—especially if you've come across popular books like *The China Study*, the 2011 documentary *Forks Over Knives*, or others in the long line of resources promoting total or near-total exclusion of animal products. According to this line of thinking, the only necessary—and appropriate—amount of animal products for the human body is zero. Welcome to the world of veganism.

As we saw earlier with Bill Clinton, a number of other famous people (who, for better or worse, are one of the best barometers of a diet's popularity) have hopped on the plant-based bandwagon.[28] But even for those deaf to celebrity endorsements, veganism seems to be gaining legitimacy as a tool for disease reversal, longevity, and overall well-being. A group of whole food, plant-based diet doctors—including John McDougall, Neal Barnard, Caldwell Esselstyn, Dean Ornish, and Joel Fuhrman—have had impressive success using their protocols to treat a variety of health conditions, most notably heart disease and diabetes.[29,30,31,32] It's no surprise, then, that such successes lend some weight to the argument that veganism—or the closest thing to it that we can muster—is the optimal diet for humans.

Unfortunately it's not quite so simple. As often happens with any switch from industrially processed products to whole, natural foods, there's more to the story than the mere elimination of animal products. All existing trials of disease-slaying vegan or near-vegan diets involve reducing or eliminating refined grain products, sugar, high fructose corn syrup, industrially processed vegetable oils, soft drinks, and most other heavily processed foods. Some, like the Lifestyle Heart Trial that put Ornish's name in the books, also include stress reduction, smoking cessation, peer support, exercise, and other modifications that have nil to do with diet. When these studies show success, it's impossible to determine which variables were the ones influencing the outcome. In a word, such studies are *confounded.*

Should We Eat Like Apes?

A common argument for choosing plants over animals comes from looking at the diet of our furry, opposable-thumbed primate cousin: the chimpanzee. Sharing about 98 percent of our DNA, chimpanzees are one of our closest genetic relatives—tied only with the fruit-noshing, free-loving, remarkably promiscuous bonobos, who make up the other half of the genus *Pan.*[33]

While a nontrivial portion of the chimp diet consists of insects, eggs, and the occasional hunted mammal, chimps certainly aren't mowing down on large quantities of meat. Indeed, the majority of their diet is plucked from trees and bushes and shrubs.

Does our own anatomy suggest similar herbivorous leanings? Some argue for a "yes." For instance, Vegsource.com—one of the world's largest and highest-trafficked vegetarian websites—cites humans' muscular lips and tongue, flattened mandibular joint, large and tightly aligned teeth, narrow esophagus, moderately acidic stomach, long small intestine, and pouched colon as evidence that we have the anatomy of a "committed" herbivore—with a gastrointestinal tract "designed for a purely plant-food diet."[34] Similar arguments abound from vegetarian authors and in other vegetarian resources, depicting the human body as a plant-powered machine that inevitably suffers if it consumes other animals.[35,36]

Yet the truth about human anatomy is far more complex. In her paper "Nutritional Characteristics of Wild Primate Foods," Katharine Milton—an anthropologist specializing in the digestive physiology and dietary habits of both human and non-human primates—outlines some of the changes we've undergone over the course of our evolution.[37] It turns out that our digestive tracts, while far from being akin to those of true carnivores, feature some adaptations that point to a likely role of meat.

Gut Feelings

According to Milton, humans *do* share some basic digestive anatomy with other primates, thanks to the beauty of our evolutionary history. Despite splitting from our last common ancestor with chimpanzees—*Hominini*—somewhere between four and seven million years ago, we have the same basic gut anatomy as the apes who still roam the jungles: a simple, moderately acidic stomach; a small intestine; a small cecum; an appendix; and a sacculated colon full of numerous, tiny pouches. With a cursory glance, the "humans should eat like the other primates" argument might seem to hold water.

But the noteworthy differences come when we look at gut proportions. As Milton explains, over half of humans' total gut volume is found in the small intestine—in sharp contrast to other apes, whose capacious colons dominate their digestive systems. In fact, in primates like chimpanzees, gorillas, and orangutans, the colon is about two to three times the size of the small intestine, while the human colon is about *half* the size of our small intestine.

So what does that mean for diet? In simple terms, a big colon is

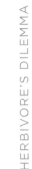

Gut Part Volume by Species

TABLE 9. Relative volume of the stomach, small intestine, cecum, and colon for six species of primate: gibbon, siamang, orangutan, gorilla, chimpanzee, and human. Humans possess notably less gut volume in the colon and more in the small intestine compared to other primates. Adapted from Dr. Katharine Milton's 1999 article, "Nutritional Characteristics of Wild Primate Foods."

good for handling "low-quality" foods like tough leaves, stems, twigs, bark, fibrous fruits, and other plant matter that requires a lot of digestive toiling to break down.

Primates that thrive on greens have a massive army of microbes in their colons that can effortlessly digest fiber and convert it into short-chain fatty acids via "hindgut fermentation"—meaning that, unlike humans, they don't choose the salad just to keep their svelte figures. Although humans have some capacity to ferment fiber in our colons and derive energy from it, we've lost the ability to do it with much efficiency. The hindgut volume in apes is around 52 percent; in humans it's shrunk to a measly 17 to 20 percent.[38] Gorillas, for instance—professional hindgut-fermenters that they are—can get a whopping 57 percent of their calories from all the fiber fermentation happening in their colons.[39] Humans would starve (or go insane from stomach gurgles) trying to do the same.

As Milton explains, humans *shouldn't* try mimicking primate diets. In her own words, "certain features of modern human gut anatomy and physiology suggest that such dietary habits probably would not now be feasible." While the dominance of the hindgut in our primate cousins suggests they're adapted to diets that are bulkier and more fibrous than what modern humans eat, our own small-intestine dominance suggests we're adapted to foods that are dense, highly digestible, and don't take a massive microbe attack to break down—such as animal products and cooked foods.

There are, of course, some remaining unknowns. When exactly in our evolutionary history did our colons become dwarfs of their ancestral selves? What provoked the human gut to change from a colon-dominated, fiber-fermenting vat of microbes capable of handling tough plant fare, to the relatively wimpy system we have now—where we need an elite diet of soft and dense foods in order to thrive? Since the earth isn't exactly littered with perfectly preserved digestive tracts from millions of years ago, it's tough to answer these questions. What we *do* know is that numerous archeological sites suggest an increasing role of animal foods, including shellfish and scavenged animals, throughout the last several million years of our history. Unlike fibrous plant matter, those foods require very little colon action and could easily have influenced its shrinkage in our modern bodies.

The evolutionary diet of humans is hard to gauge anatomically for two other reasons as well. For one, our digestive systems have—in some sense—atrophied due to our reliance on cooking and external processing to "pre-digest" the things we eat, whether those foods come from the plant or animal kingdom. (Even in those barbaric days before the George Foreman Grill and Vitamix, we at least had fire pits and hammerstones.) And secondly, we've co-evolved with tools to such a degree that we've rendered claws, tails, and sharp teeth nearly useless, making these ineffectual markers for discerning our dietary adaptations.

Despite the remaining questions, though, it's pretty clear that we can't draw a dietary parallel between humans and our primate relatives based on our digestive anatomy. Simply put, we humans cannot subsist on leaf and twig alone.

What's Missing?

On paper, meeting your nutritional needs without animal products seems simple enough. More dark, leafy greens for calcium. Fortified foods or supplements for B12. Sunshine for vitamin D. Maybe some flaxseed for those essential fatty acids. Even from mainstream sources, we're often told that's the gist of what it takes to stay healthy on a diet free from (or at least very low in) animal-based foods—and as long as we meet our nutrient targets on paper, we're good to go. In practice, though, the nutritional adequacy of veganism is neither clear-cut nor universal.

The reason some people seem to thrive on plant-based cuisines while others struggle has much to do with our fabulous diversity—particularly how we metabolize and convert plant-based nutrients, a fate resting largely in the hands of genetics (go ahead and blame your parents for that one). Here's a rundown of the nutrients some portion of the population will struggle to glean from plant foods alone.

Vitamin A: This nutrient is one of the biggest potential absentees as far as plant-based diets go. But what about carrots, sweet potatoes, and leafy greens, you ask? It's actually a popular misconception that these plant-based foods are vitamin A powerhouses.

"True" vitamin A exists only in animal foods. Plants, on the other hand, feature an array of *carotenoids*, more than six hundred different types, of which about fifty, including beta-carotene, will convert to the usable form of vitamin A in your body. Well, at least in theory.

Here's the problem: the carotenoid-to-vitamin-A conversion rates vary tremendously from person to person, and not everyone can squeeze enough vitamin A out of plant foods to stay healthy. Some folks inherit gene alleles that dramatically reduce the body's ability to convert carotenoids, and in other cases, problems such as liver diseases, food allergies, celiac disease, parasite infection, *H. pylori* infection, and deficiencies in iron or zinc can put a major damper on the carotenoid conversion process.[40] As a result, good converters of carotenoids might breeze through a plant-based diet with no vitamin A troubles, whereas a poor converter may experience a gradual onset of deficiency symptoms—often beginning with skin problems, poor night vision, and infertility.

Vitamin B12: Despite the occasional rumor to the contrary, there are no reliable, naturally occurring sources of vitamin B12 in plants. Some seaweeds, commonly mis-cited as bestowers of B12, actually contain B12 *analogues* that won't actually improve your true B12 status.[41] But virtually every study conducted on the subject shows that vegans experience much higher rates of B12 deficiency than omnivores or vegetarians, and have elevated homocysteine as a result, which increases blood clotting and may raise your risk of heart disease. In fact, low B12 and high homocysteine may very well have contributed to the early demise of prominent vegans like H. Jay Dinshah and T.C. Fry, both long-term adherents of their vegan diets who passed away before their time.

Vitamin K2: Although it tends to get lumped in with vitamin K1 with regrettable frequency, vitamin K2 is in a class of its own. Woefully unknown to the public and mainstream health experts alike, vitamin K2 is critical for a healthy heart and skeleton, working synergistically with other fat-soluble vitamins and some minerals.

Among other things, it helps shuttle calcium out of your arteries (where it contributes to plaque formation) and into your bones and teeth, where it rightfully belongs. Unlike vitamin K1, which is abundant in some vegan foods like dark leafy greens, vitamin K2 is only found in certain bacteria and animal products such as dairy (especially hard cheeses and butter), organ meats, eggs, and fish eggs. The only abundant vegan source is *natto*—a not-always-appetizing fermented soybean product that contains K2-producing bacteria. Other fermented vegetable products, like sauerkraut, can contain some K2 depending on the type of bacteria they contain.

Omega-3 fats, docosahexaenoic acid (DHA), and eicosapentaenoic acid (EPA): If you're a vegan, your main source of these essential fatty acids is through your body's conversion of their precursor, alpha-linolenic acid (ALA). However, a number of dietary and genetic factors influence how well your body makes that conversion—leaving the potential for DHA and EPA insufficiency, even if you have a decent intake of ALA from flaxseed and other vegan foods.

Should We Jump on the Starch Wagon?

The hallmark of many plant-based diets is not just the acceptance of starch, but the warm embrace of all things whole-grainy and tuberous. In fact, the pro-starch message is reverberating loudly outside the walls of the USDA, entering the realm of esteemed plant-based diet doctors like Dr. John McDougall. But America's amber waves are no joke.

While a boon for many farmers (and, in its current subsidy-soaked state, the economy), this advice sweeps individual starch tolerance under the rug, with tragic consequences. Just as Luise Light predicted many years ago, a mass prescription of starch-centrism for the country has failed to restore America's health, especially when guidelines are so lenient with "junk" carbohydrates. Obesity and diabetes have only continued to soar. And vegetarianism—as it's typically practiced today—tends to share the USDA pyramid's unconditional emphasis on grains, often flying its starch emphasis under the banner of healthfulness.

While some people may thrive on a diet higher in starch, mounting research shows that it wreaks havoc for others. And the evidence is far beyond anecdotal. It turns out some of us are genetically blessed with better starch tolerance than others—a fact that should be acknowledged in any guideline that tries to steer us toward good health. When it comes to vegetarian eating in particular, the narrower range of food groups can lead to an even greater emphasis on starches.

Starchivores and Starchiphobes: A Journey Through Your Genetic Innards

Your saliva might seem uneventful and slimy, but it's actually a pretty happening place. In fact, it's teeming with all sorts of proteins that kick off the digestion process—including *alpha-amylase,* an enzyme that breaks down starch into sugar. If you've ever held a cracker or piece of bread in your mouth and witnessed it miraculously turn sweet, that was your amylase in action, chopping up all those bland starch molecules into tasty sugars. (Even after you swallow, amylase remains hard at work: partially digested starch protects amylase from getting deactivated by your stomach acid, so any amylase-riddled globs of potato, rice, noodles, or other starchy foods you've chewed up can continue their journey onto becoming sugar molecules even after entering your belly.[42])

In order to furnish the mouth with starch-digesting proteins, we all carry copies of a gene called AMY1, which encodes the salivary amylase enzyme. Indeed, amylase is a gem some plant-based diet advocates cite as evidence for a starchy diet being optimal for mankind. In his book *The Starch Solution,* McDougall discusses human amylase status as evidence that we are, as a species, genetic starchivores:

> Studies of the gene [AMY1] coding for amylase ... found that humans have on average six copies of the gene compared to two copies in other, "lesser" primates. This difference means that human saliva produces six to eight times more of the starch-digesting enzyme amylase.... It was our ability to digest and meet our energy needs with starch that allowed us to migrate north and south and inhabit the entire planet.[43]

Just one problem: it's not that simple. It turns out the number of AMY1 copies contained in our genes is not the same for everyone. And the amount of salivary amylase we produce is tightly correlated to the number of AMY1 copies we inherited. In humans, AMY1 copy number can range from one to fifteen, and amylase levels in saliva can range from barely detectable to 50 percent of the saliva's total protein.[44] That's a *lot* of variation!

Where you land on the amylase spectrum is more than just luck of the draw, too. Folks from traditionally starch-centric populations, like the Japanese or the Hazda of Tanzania, tend to carry more copies of AMY1 than folks from low-starch-eating populations, like Siberian pastoralists or hunter-gatherers from the Congo rainforest.[45] One analysis found that nearly twice as many people from high-starch populations carried six or more copies of AMY1 (considered the average number for humans) compared to folks from low-starch populations.[46] Since AMY1 copy number varies greatly among different groups within the same region, it's clear that traditional diet has a greater influence on this gene than simple geography.

The reason for such vast variation is rooted in the nutritional pressures that clobbered us throughout history. For populations whose food staples were starches, such as roots and tubers and grains, carrying more copies of AMY1—and packing more amylase in their saliva as a result—would have been a major boon for survival. Those best able to metabolize starches, in those cases, would be the healthiest and strongest. Their genes would muscle their way into dominance.

On the flip side, populations relying more on animal foods and non-starchy carbohydrates from fruit, honey, or milk wouldn't face much selective pressure for amylase production. In those populations, folks with less starch-digesting power would be at no disadvantage to those with more. Those with fewer copies of AMY1 would remain warmly embraced in the gene pool, with other adaptive pressures taking precedence over starch tolerance.

The same pattern holds true for our closest genetic relatives. Non-human primates that rely on starchy plant matter produce significantly more amylase than species like the chimpanzee and bonobo, who favor ripe, low-starch fruit.[47,48] As a result, chimpanzees universally carry only two copies of AMY1, and the closely related bonobos all carry four—similar to humans from starch-sparse populations.[49]

What's more, the lack of variation in gene copy number in all primates except humans emphasizes the quirkiness of our diet history. While other primates embrace a pretty consistent menu within their species, humans have endured impressive dietary diversity since we've split from our last common primate ancestor—a legacy that's stamped its mark all over our genome.

So what happens when low amylase producers encounter, say, a heaping pile of pasta? Do their bodies simply escort it out like an ID-checking bouncer at a club, throwing it back from whence it came before it can do any damage? Not quite. It turns out that for folks without amylase-supercharged saliva, feasting on starch might have dire consequences for blood sugar and insulin levels—calling into question the USDA's wisdom in prescribing a starch-based diet for the entire nation.

Researchers at the Monell Chemical Senses Center in Philadelphia wanted to learn why and conducted a groundbreaking trial on starch tolerance.[50] Their study looked at blood sugar and insulin responses to starch consumption among high-amylase producers versus their low-amylase counterparts—the first time anyone had actually investigated whether there might be a difference. The participants were all healthy, normal-weight, mixed-race adults with significantly higher or lower salivary amylase than average.

Each subject came into the laboratory twice, for two different feedings: one using 50 grams of pure glucose and the other using 50 grams of cornstarch hydrolysate. After each session, the participants hung around for two hours and had their blood sugar and insulin levels monitored. As seemed logical, the researchers thought the high-amylase participants would have the strongest blood sugar response from eating starch, seeing as they'd be breaking it down into sugar molecules more efficiently.

But the human body, the infinite wonderland that it is, had a surprise in store, and the study took a fascinating turn. The results—published in the *Journal of Nutrition* in 2012—showed that low-amylase producers faced skyrocketing blood sugar after eating starch, in contrast to the less dramatic rise seen among high-amylase producers. The paper included a graph capturing the trend. (See Table 10.)

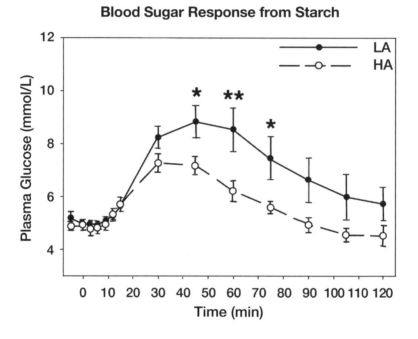

Blood Sugar Response from Starch

TABLE 10. This table shows the differences in blood sugar (plasma glucose) levels after consuming pure starch for low amylase producers (LA) versus high amylase producers (HA).

After about fifteen minutes, the low-amylase group (represented by the top line with black dots) started leaving the high-amylase group in the dust, at least as far as blood sugar was concerned. Not only did their levels peak at about 2 mmol/L (or 36 mg/dL) greater than the high amylase group, but the profound difference continued all the way to the end of the two-hour monitoring phase, and likely persisted well beyond that. Simply put, the low-amylase group's blood sugar rose higher and *stayed* higher for a shockingly long time.

When the procedure was repeated using glucose, though, the results were a different story. Folks with low amylase levels saw an overall milder response than they did with starch—with blood sugar dropping back to normal levels more quickly and not diverging much from the high-amylase group. If anything, that suggests low-amylase producers might actually have better tolerance of sugar than they do of starch—a conclusion that could and *should* send shockwaves through modern dietary recommendations that tend to treat sugar as the only offensive carb of the bunch while hurling starch atop a high and mighty throne.

Can you see why crowning starch as king of the food groups has likely done immeasurable damage to our health? Even today, half of our grain intake comes from refined sources per USDA guidelines. And the people who come up on the short end of the breadstick are are the low-amylase producers.

In fact, the study's researchers warn that such individuals "may be at greater risk for insulin resistance and diabetes if chronically ingesting starch-rich diets"—raising the possibility that AMY1 gene copy may play a role in who succumbs to obesity and diabetes and who is graciously spared. And if that's the case, perhaps AMY1 should be considered an important new risk factor for such conditions. The researchers even proposed putting the study's findings into clinical use by screening individuals for low AMY1 gene copy number, thus equipping patients with knowledge about their risk—and hopefully thwarting disease before it strikes.

We haven't pinpointed when exactly our ancestors started accumulating more AMY1 copies and revving up their starch-metabolizing capabilities. But the adaptation may be at least partially grain related—especially seeing as agricultural populations universally carry AMY1 copy numbers on the higher end of the spectrum. (Prior to domesticating grains, humans may have started facing selective pressure for AMY1 with the control of fire—at which point hard, starchy, barely edible roots and tubers could be softened with heat and turned into exciting new calorie sources.)

For Americans struggling to conform to dietary guidelines in order to boost their health (as well as vegetarians embracing a similarly starch-centric pyramid), the amylase issue spells trouble in a big way. Imagine entering a rowing race where half of the participants can use oars and half must paddle wildly with their hands. It wouldn't be long before wails of unfairness echoed through the crowd and riots ensued, right? Being a high-amylase producer offers a similar game-changing advantage, at least when the waters we're sculling through are filled with starch. In a population where some people have nearly eight times as many AMY1 copies as others, and saliva can range from amylase-replete to amylase-barren, prescribing a starchy diet to the entire population is a recipe for disaster. Those at a metabolic disadvantage will always be left flailing near the shore, unable to keep pace with the rest. By ignoring individual variation regarding starch tolerance, promoters of high-starch diets for every human being do our collective health a disservice.

The Best of Both Worlds

They say imitation is the sincerest form of flattery, so hopefully the vegetarian movement will feel honored when omnivores skim some of the pro-health foam off the top of vegetarianism without going as far as totally avoiding meat. Here are a few tips:

- Make the plant-based portion of your diet full of whole, fresh, minimally processed produce. The marvelous thing about many plant foods—especially the fibrous-vegetable kind—is that they're low in energy density, meaning you can pile them onto your plate without having to swap out other delicious things. Avoid "empty," denser foods like bread, sugar, pastries, pasta, and other items that deliver less nutrition with more calories.

- Cut down on the forms of meat with known mechanisms for contributing to disease—namely well-done meat, or anything that's touched open fire via grilling or other high-temperature cooking. As we learned in the *Meet Your Meat* chapter, these foods contain compounds that can act as carcinogens in the human body. Stick to gently cooked meats, and favor cooking methods like steaming, stewing, and baking.

- Aim for nutrient density. Rock stars of the plant world include dark leafy greens, brightly colored vegetables, mushrooms, berries, seaweeds, and fermented vegetables. And for animal foods, that includes organ meats like liver, bivalves like oysters and clams, eggs, fish roe, cod liver oil, and raw dairy from pastured cows.

- Act like a vegetarian. In perhaps unfairly stereotypical terms, that means being more physically active, abstaining from smoking, watching the number of margaritas you slam back, and generally being a health-conscious, functioning member of society.

STAYING HEALTHY WHEN
ANIMAL FOODS ARE OFF THE MENU

As a former decade-long vegetarian, I understand and respect that food choices are sometimes based on more than our own health—and while this book doesn't promote plant-only diets as an optimal choice for the human body, there are certainly ways to make the best out of a meatless, eggless, and dairyless situation. If you're personally committed to abstaining from animal products, here are some tips for maximizing your chances of staying healthy.

1. *Enhance your beta-carotene absorption and conversion.* Vitamin A insufficiency can be a big problem for folks who don't convert carotenoids very well. To boost your absorption and conversion capacity, couple beta-carotene rich foods (like carrots, sweet potatoes, and dark leafy greens) with a source of fat, such as olive oil or avocado slices on a salad. Likewise, identify and treat any health problems that can disturb your gut ecology and hinder carotenoid absorption, including food allergies, celiac disease, parasite infections, or low stomach acid. And finally, lightly cook some of your orange or yellow vegetables to break down their fiber and give your body better access to their nutritional bounty.

2. *Supplement with a vegan form of Vitamin D3.*

3. *Supplement with vitamin B12.* The standard recommendation is to take about 10 mcgs a day, or 2000 mcgs once per week.

4. *Supplement with vitamin K2 or make natto a regular part of your menu.*

5. *Keep your thyroid in good shape.* Health-conscious vegans may unintentionally wind up with two strikes against their thyroid gland: lack of iodine (either from cutting back on salt or switching from iodized salt to natural sea salt), and a menu packed with so-called "goitrogenic" vegetables like kale, broccoli, cauliflower, and cabbage, which can interfere with thyroid function in certain contexts. The best whole-food vegan source of iodine is seaweed—particularly dulse, kelp, and alaria. And as far as goitrogenic veggies go, they're unlikely to induce thyroid problems at normal levels of consumption (and they have some great anti-cancer compounds that make them a lovely addition to your diet in general). But if you have any preexisting thyroid diseases or iodine deficiency, be sure to moderate your intake.

6. *Maximize your iron absorption.* Especially if you're a pre-menopausal woman, combining iron-rich plant foods (like dark greens) with something high in vitamin C (like citrus) helps enhance your absorption of nonheme iron.

7. *Avoid high omega-6 vegetable oils and supplement with vegan DHA.* Without seafood as an omega-3 fallback, vegan diets can tilt toward an unhealthy ratio of omega-6 to omega-3 fats. To remedy that, avoid omega-6-rich vegetable oils like soybean oil, corn oil, cottonseed oil, sunflower oil, and margarines made from these oils, and opt for coconut oil, olive oil, macadamia nut oil, or red palm oil. Likewise, you can increase omega-3 intake by supplementing with a vegan source of DHA, or by consuming unheated, ground chia seeds, hemp seeds, or flaxseeds.

8. *Limit your intake of imitation meats and other heavily processed vegan foods.*

9. *Properly prepare any legumes, grains, or nuts you eat.* These foods contain phytates, which block the absorption of calcium and iron and other minerals. They also feature enzyme inhibitors and tannins that can cause digestive distress. If you choose to include legumes, grains, or nuts in your diet, you can neutralize some of their troublesome components and increase mineral availability by first soaking them in warm water and an acidic medium (like vinegar) for at least seven hours in the case of grains and nuts, and twenty-four hours in the case of legumes. Then rinse and cook as usual.

10. **If comfortable ethically, consider adding oysters or other non-sentient bivalves to your diet.** Along with being some of the most nutrient-dense foods in existence, bivalves (such as clams and oysters) lack a central nervous system, placing them—in some sense—in a limbo between the plant kingdom and animal kingdom. Depending on your reasons for being vegan, they can be an excellent way to fill in some of the nutritional gaps present in plant-only diets.

NEW GEOMETRY

12
A Future
Informed by the Past

Now that we've determined what *doesn't* work, it's time to piece together what *does*. Unless we learn to live off photosynthesis and do away with the need for food entirely, we can't slam a wrecking ball against the Food Guide Pyramid without constructing something new in its rubbled place.

But what we need *isn't* another set of one-size-fits-all guidelines, a pyramid or plate or dodecahedron illustrating oversimplified rules for a theoretical public. We don't need more advice based on faceless averages and political nannying. We don't need another dietary death star pointing its super laser at rivaling paradigms. What we need is an approach to diet that synthesizes what has worked—scientifically, historically, globally, *consistently*—and pairs it with the reality of individual variation. And that means looking at all the successes out there and finding what they have in common. What universal themes emerge when we step back and view the bigger picture? What can we distill from the chaos?

Without forgetting our goal to transcend the pyramid paradigm altogether, let's start by touring some popular, purportedly health-boosting diets and seeing where they intersect. In this chapter, we'll be gleaning the underlying wisdom from our current body of knowledge and exploring how to apply it to your own life.

Modern Trinity:
Paleo, Mediterranean & Whole-Foods, Plant-Based

While the sea of popular diets is teeming with more options than ever before, three in particular have bubbled to the top with the promise of not only stripping away excess pounds, but also combating chronic disease (and all manner of other ills) in the process. Those contenders are the Paleolithic-style diets (and their dairy-loving cousin, Primal), the Mediterranean diet, and the whole-foods, plant-based diets.

As a perfect example of why the public is mired in confusion, the three eating programs may seem as different as night, day, and the Twilight Zone at first glance—yet they all seem to produce glowing successes, positive health outcomes, and equally fervent groups of devotees. In health debates, they're often pitted against one another, gladiator fight-to-the-death style, with a satisfying victor rarely emerging. So what lessons can they collectively teach us?

To answer that question, let's first glance at the spec sheets for each of these diets in case you're not yet familiar with them.

Ancestral, Paleolithic-style Diets

The details: Under the premise that human genetics (and our evolutionarily sculpted nutritional requirements) have changed little since the dawn of agriculture, Paleolithic-style diets, sometimes referred to as "ancestral eating," emphasize foods available during the Paleolithic era:

- Animals from both land and sea
- Eggs
- Vegetables
- Tubers
- Low-glycemic fruits such as berries (with higher sugar varieties like pineapples and mangos sometimes limited)
- Nuts and seeds
- Animal fats like tallow and lard

The Primal Blueprint offers more flexibility, especially in the way that dairy (full-fat, high-quality products) get a stamp of approval, as do "sensible indulgences" such as dark chocolate and red wine. Other paleo-inspired variations, such as the Perfect Health Diet, allow Neolithic foods like white rice. Generally, with all the Paleolithic-style diets, there's an emphasis on pasture-raised meats and organic, locally grown plant foods. Cold-pressed, low-PUFA oils like olive oil and coconut oil also get a free pass.

The claim to fame: Along with tidal waves of anecdotal success, research on paleo-style diets—although mostly comprised of smaller, short-term studies at this point—has generally been promising. The pool of current studies gives a bow to paleo for improving glucose control, insulin levels, triglycerides, HDL cholesterol, blood pressure, body weight, BMI, and satiety.[1,2,3,4,5]

The caveats: The Paleolithic-style diets existing in scientific studies and the Paleolithic diet existing in practice are apparently two different beasts. Real-world paleo—per the guidance of popular diet and recipe books—tends to embrace animal fats like tallow and lard, fatty cuts of meat, coconut oil, and other unabashedly high-fat fare. Yet if you follow the golden research rule of reading the fine print, you'll notice that the paleo-style menus used in studies are almost always comprised of lean meats and limited oils, if the latter is used at all. The result is a surprisingly low fat intake, sometimes even lower than the USDA's recommendations. (For instance, one under-the-paleo-umbrella study led by researcher Kerin O'Dea—in which diabetic Australian Aborigines returned to a traditional hunter-gatherer diet for seven weeks—averaged only 13 percent of calories from fat, due to the leanness of wild game.[6]) That discrepancy makes it hard to extrapolate the existing research done on Paleolithic diets to the form they take in practice, and highlights the need for longer-term, larger studies using a more liberal intake of paleo-friendly fats.

In addition, some tenets of paleo—such as the avoidance of legumes—are based more on theory than clinical evidence. And as we saw in the *Meet your Meat* chapter, problems may arise in Paleolithic diets tilted too far in favor of muscle meat while neglecting other parts of the animal. There's also some evidence that we *have* adapted, to varying degrees, to foods introduced more recently in our evolution, including through changes in our gut biome.[7]

ANCESTRAL, PALEOLITHIC-STYLE DIETS

A FUTURE INFORMED BY THE PAST

Paleo Autoimmune emphasizes gut health and is the most restrictive, shunning edible nightshades such as potatoes, tomatoes, eggplant, and peppers.

The Perfect Health Diet embraces "safe starches" low in antinutrients, including white rice, tapioca, taro, and potatoes.

The Primal Blueprint offers the most flexibility, allowing for full-fat, high-quality dairy and "sensible indulgences" such as dark chocolate and wine. It also emphasizes healthy lifestyle habits such as sunlight, sleep, play, community, and nature immersion.

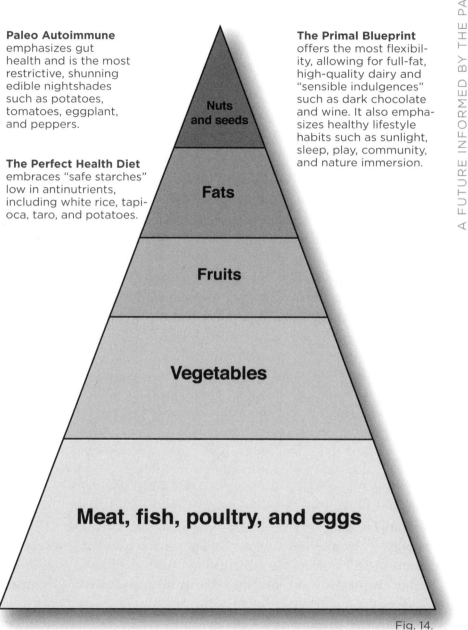

Nuts and seeds

Fats

Fruits

Vegetables

Meat, fish, poultry, and eggs

Fig. 14.

Paleolithic-style diets shun grains and legumes and come in several flavors: Paleo, Primal Blueprint, Perfect Health Diet, and Paleo-Autoimmune, among others. In most cases, meat consumes the bulk of dietary calories, not the majority of space on your plate.

The Mediterranean Diet

The details: First inspired by the dazzling health exhibited on the Greek isle of Crete and popularized by Ancel Keys, the Mediterranean diet—as it's portrayed in our modern diet culture—emphasizes abundant plant foods in the form of whole grains, fresh fruit, fresh vegetables, legumes, nuts and seeds, and generous use of olive oil, along with moderate amounts of dairy products, fish, and poultry. Red meat and eggs can sneak onto the plate only occasionally.

The claim to fame: Since hopping the pond from Europe to American dieters, the Mediterranean way of eating has gathered an impressive entourage of clinical studies in its favor—suggesting the diet can improve blood lipids, insulin resistance, metabolic syndrome, antioxidant capacity, and even cut heart disease rates and cancer in certain individuals.[13] But it earned its first, and biggest, gold star by promoting spectacular health on the epidemiological front. The Mediterranean diet practiced in Crete has been linked to fabulous longevity, enough to land it on the "Blue Zone" reserved for areas with unusually long life spans.[14]

The caveats: Modern interpretations of the Mediterranean-diet-formerly-known-as-the-Cretan-diet tend to overlook (or downright convolute) some of the most important aspects of the region's eating habits. Among the long-living Cretans, snails—rich in omega-3 fats, iron, copper, magnesium, selenium, and other health-promoting goodies—are an important mainstay rarely mentioned in pop diet books preaching the Mediterranean cuisine. Likewise, Cretans rely heavily on wild edible greens, many of which put our store-bought vegetables to shame in terms of spectacular nutritional content and antioxidant activity.[15,16,17] (The variety, too, is noteworthy: Greek cuisine makes use of over 150 wild vegetable species.[18]) Fasting, as we saw in an earlier chapter, is also widespread due to the prevalence of Orthodox Christianity in Crete.

Moreover, while our modern snail-free, fasting-free interpretation of the Mediterranean diet tends to fare well compared to "standard" diets featuring more processed foods, it doesn't always emerge victorious when pitted against other specialized eating plans. One study evaluating the effects of a Mediterranean diet versus a Paleolithic-style diet on glucose tolerance found that the latter produced significantly better outcomes.[19]

THE MEDITERRANEAN DIET

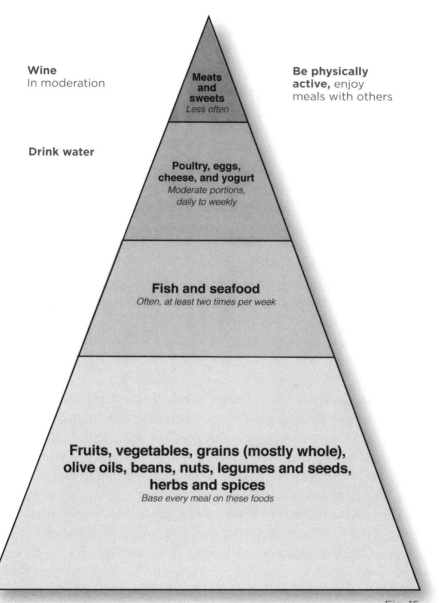

Wine
In moderation

Drink water

Be physically active, enjoy meals with others

Meats and sweets
Less often

Poultry, eggs, cheese, and yogurt
Moderate portions, daily to weekly

Fish and seafood
Often, at least two times per week

Fruits, vegetables, grains (mostly whole), olive oils, beans, nuts, legumes and seeds, herbs and spices
Base every meal on these foods

A FUTURE INFORMED BY THE PAST

Fig. 15.

The Mediterranean diet diverges from the lowfat message by making liberal use of olive oil. The Mediterranean paradigm also advocates regular exercise and mindful eating—that is, taking time to enjoy your meal, preferably with others.

Whole-Foods, Plant-based Diets

The details: Most forms of whole-food, plant-based eating—including the programs recommended by John McDougall, Neal Barnard, Caldwell Esselstyn, and Dean Ornish—center on unprocessed starches including potatoes, sweet potatoes, whole grains, squash, legumes, and various root vegetables, along with a spectrum of non-starchy vegetables and some fruit. Plant-based-diet advocate Joel Fuhrman allows more in the way of fat from whole-food sources such as nuts.

The claim to fame: Whole-food, plant-based diets have enjoyed a fair amount of clinical success when it comes to treating heart disease, diabetes, and possibly other chronic conditions. Both Esselstyn and Ornish have helped patients halt and even reverse heart disease through strict adherence to their programs (though Ornish's includes more changes than just a diet overhaul).[8,9] In diabetics, Neal Barnard's work suggests very lowfat vegan diets are more effective at reducing weight and improving blood lipids than standard diabetes diets.[10]

Additional studies show plant-based cuisines could have a beneficial effect on rheumatoid arthritis, although those particular chunks of research are confounded by the diets also being gluten-free and integrating fasting.[11,12]

The caveats: Whole-food, plant-based diets appear promising for treating some chronic conditions when they are compared to the highly processed standard American diet. But diets that nearly or completely eliminate animal products are—right now—experiments in the sense that no known human population has lived exclusively on plant foods and thrived. They operate on the assumption that we've not only identified every nutrient necessary for the human body (and understand how they interact), but that we can adequately replace those derived from animals with plant-based versions. Such diets need to be monitored for their long-term effects on fertility, bone development, and other issues associated with lack of fat-soluble vitamins and other nutrients. Many of those problems might not crop up for decades, or even until the next generation is born and develops. As we've seen in previous chapters, animal foods have been falsely accused in many cases, and eating "nose to tail" while also being mindful of gentler cooking methods can resolve most (if not all) of the problems potentially associated with animal foods.

WHOLE-FOODS, PLANT-BASED DIETS

High-fat whole foods
such as avocadoes, nuts, olives;
whole food-sweetened treats;
dairy substitutes such as oat,
almond, rice, and soy milk.
Use sparingly

Joel Fuhrman's
"Nutritarian" diet focuses
on nutrient density and
allows more nuts, seeds,
and avocados than
lower-fat plant-based
programs. It also limits
starchy foods like grains
and potatoes.

**Leafy, green
vegetables**
such as collards,
spinach, and kale. Eat
at least 2-3 servings
(1 cup raw or 1/2 cup
cooked) per day

Legumes
(beans, peas, lentils
and seeds)
Consume 2-3 servings
(1/2 cup cooked
legumes or
1 Tbsp seeds) every day

Whole grains
such as brown rice, barley, quinoa,
oats, amaranth, whole wheat, whole
grain pasta, and sprouted grains.
6-11 servings (1/2 cup cooked or
1 slice whole grain bread) daily

Fruit (all types)
Consume 2-4 servings
(1 piece or 1/2 cup)
every day

Vegetables
(all types,
including starchy)
Eat as much and
as many different colors
as possible each day

**Drink plenty of pure water every day.
Exercise at least 1 hour every day**

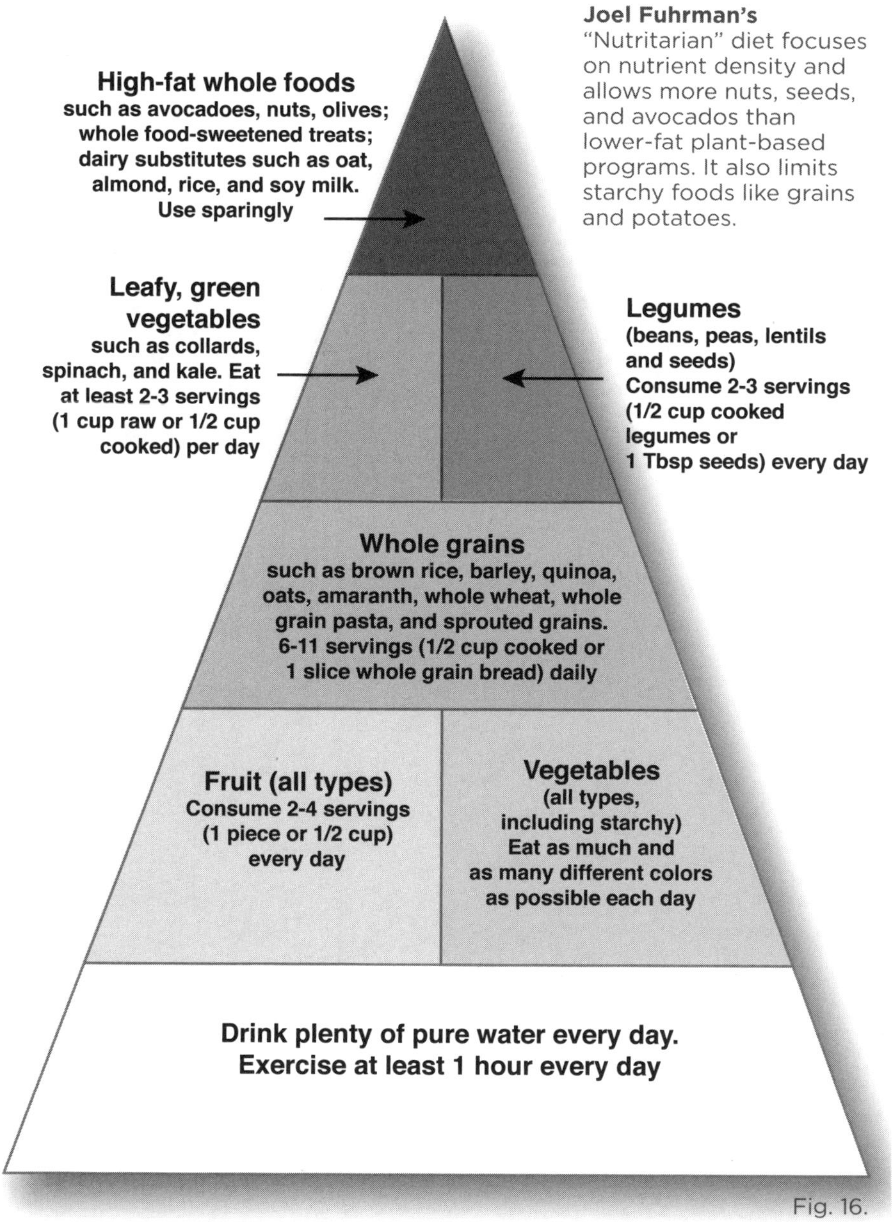

Fig. 16.

Whole-foods, plant-based diets emphasize minimally processed grains, legumes, fruits, vegetables, herbs, and spices. Along with reducing or eliminating animal products, most keep fat intake very low, shunning oils and high-fat plant foods like nuts and avocados.

Where Do They Intersect?

At this point, you might be wondering how it's possible for three very different diets to all claim some success. It's like an Escher drawing: fascinating, but fundamentally inscrutable. Fear not—we're about to blast away the confusion. For starters, we can look at dietary themes in two different ways: the process of accumulation and the process of elimination.

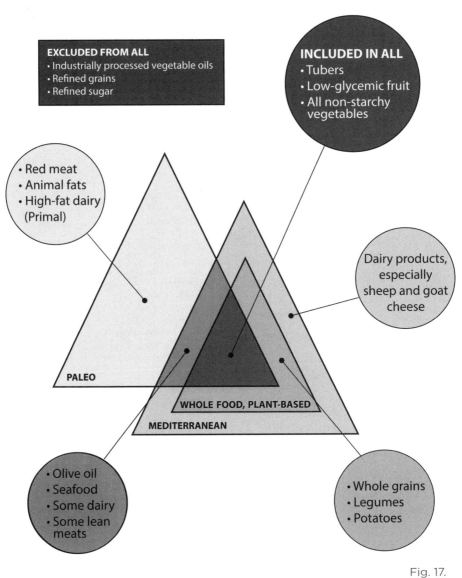

EXCLUDED FROM ALL
- Industrially processed vegetable oils
- Refined grains
- Refined sugar

INCLUDED IN ALL
- Tubers
- Low-glycemic fruit
- All non-starchy vegetables

- Red meat
- Animal fats
- High-fat dairy (Primal)

Dairy products, especially sheep and goat cheese

PALEO

WHOLE FOOD, PLANT-BASED

MEDITERRANEAN

- Olive oil
- Seafood
- Some dairy
- Some lean meats

- Whole grains
- Legumes
- Potatoes

Fig. 17.

Accumulation asks: *What do these health-promoting diets all seem to include?* On the surface, it doesn't look like much: vegetables and tubers make the cut, and that's about it (though the tubers might get nixed on the very low-carb versions of a Paleolithic-style diet, so they're on the fence).

But elimination asks: *What do these health-promoting diets all seem to omit?* Here's where it starts to make more sense. From this angle, the answer is a surprisingly consistent list of offenders—as the Paleolithic-style diets, the plant-based diets, and the Mediterranean diet all shun many of the same items:

- Refined flour
- Refined sugar
- Industrially processed vegetable oils
- Chemical preservatives and lab-produced anythings
- Nearly any creation coming in a crinkly tinfoil package, a micro-wavable tray, or a McDonald's takeout bag

As you can see, **all three of our diet gladiators kick modern, heavily processed fare to the curb**. Could their shared list of black-listed foods be responsible, at least in part, for their similar successes with health promotion and weight loss? In this case, perhaps it really is about what we *don't* eat as much as what we do.

Now let's crank it up a notch. Look back at the caveats of each of these diets for a moment. Notice that none of them, at least as they are popularly implemented, have been eaten in a real-world setting across a span of generations. The Paleolithic-style diets are an approximation of our ancestral eating habits, but they have to fill our anthropological knowledge gaps with patches of guesswork. As for the plant-based diets, contrary to what followers may claim, no documented society has permanently eliminated all animal products (and lived to tell about it). And the Mediterranean diet misses some important elements of its original namesake cuisine. A more valuable comparison, then, might be the traditional diets that *have* been, until recent decades, the mainstay of actual human communities for time immemorial. And lucky for us, we have some examples of exactly that.

Weston A. Price
and Nature's Great Biological Laboratory

Perhaps our best clues about universal themes in diets that promote extraordinary health come from an unlikely man: a globetrotting dentist named Weston A. Price.

As a dentist, Price had a unique, from-the-mouth-side-out perspective of the health decline rapidly gripping America. When he'd first started his practice in the late 1800s, the teeth landing beneath his dental probe had been in pretty good shape. But within a single generation, his younger patients began to show the signs of full-blown tooth decay, "squished" dental arches, and teeth jutting waywardly out of their sockets instead of growing in straight. (The *dental arch*, by the way, is the curve of each jaw that holds your teeth.) And to make matters worse, Price noticed that poor dental health seemed to go hand-in-hand with other forms of "physical degeneration." As he put it: "The folks with cavities and malformed dental arches were also suffering from disease or general weakness elsewhere in their bodies." It was a mystery Price felt compelled to solve—a prelude to later big-hitters like Keys and Yudkin, who chased the trail of physical decline through the heart rather than the mouth.

In an era before fat (or any other singled-out nutrient) was considered a dietary evil, Price took a more global approach, quite literally. Though he began his quest in the lab—spending twenty-five years conducting animal studies on tooth decay while serving as the director of the American Dental Association's Research Institute—he eventually expanded his scope to living humans. His animal research had convinced him that some sort of "protective" substances were missing from modern menus, though he couldn't identify at the time what those might be. And he realized that instead of studying sick people to find out what they were doing wrong, he ought to study healthy people to find out what they were doing right. Such individuals would serve as a sort of natural control, a *standard of excellence* to see just how superb the human body could be.

There was just one problem: America was plumb out of its stock of "healthy people." Pristine mouths were few and far between, and other forms of disease—both infectious and degenerative—were rampant. In order to find truly robust human specimens, Price would need to look elsewhere. Tens of thousands of miles elsewhere, in fact.

PREGNANCY CLUES

It's worth mentioning that most of Price's groups had, in addition to their traditional fare, special foods or diets fed to women before and during pregnancy (and sometimes to men prior to conception), as well as cultural rules about "spacing" between pregnancies in order for the body to replete its stores before the next round of baby-making. It makes sense, actually: you wouldn't embark on a road trip without making sure your car was full of gas, or go for a long hike without stocking your backpack with plenty of food to sustain you. Likewise, the healthiest natives knew that pregnancy—an experience demanding a great deal of the body's resources—would produce the hardiest babies when women had enough nutritional stores to support two lives at once.

For the coastal groups with access to sea life, pre-pregnancy eating universally included fish eggs and often shellfish. Pastoral communities relied on dairy products from cows eating rapidly growing grass, as the resulting butter fat was highest in nutrients. In Africa, some tribes gathered certain plants from swamps and marshes and streams, favoring in particular one called water hyacinth. These were dried and burned, and the ashes were added to mothers' food as a supplement.

Collectively, Price's findings suggest we may not place enough importance on preconception nutrition—and that the health of children depends not only on what they eat, but also on what their mothers ate before even becoming pregnant.

"A comprehensive study of modern degeneration will require the use of controls," he wrote in his 1939 book *Nutrition and Physical Degeneration,* the crowning jewel of his career. Not finding such controls in his own country, he explained, "It became necessary to look elsewhere in Nature's great biological laboratory, which has been in operation through the history of life."[20] That search led him and his wife everywhere from the parched lands of Africa to the frigid Arctic North, all on a quest to find populations spared from the health decline of the industrialized world.

And in these unperturbed pockets of the planet, where humans lived and ate as their ancestors had done for generations, that's exactly what he found. Groups of remote hunter-gatherers, pastoralists, horticulturists, and agriculturists—all united by their breathtakingly good health.

Along with performing extensive dental exams, Price took thousands of photographs of the people he encountered, gathered detailed data about their diets, investigated hospitals, queried community doctors, searched for signs of disease, and collected samples of local foods and soil to analyze. Not only were those populations virtually free from dental problems—with perfectly straight teeth and cavity-free mouths, despite most of them never touching a toothbrush in their lives—but they also seemed protected from other chronic diseases overtaking American bodies. As Price described,

> Associated with a fine physical condition the isolated primitive groups have a high level of immunity to many of our modern degenerative processes, including tuberculosis, arthritis, heart disease, and affections of the internal organs.[21]

And it wasn't just that the groups had won the genetic lottery, either. Price's health-hunt included another layer as well, one that distinguished his work from other observational studies and made his research utterly invaluable. He specifically sought out groups that could be closely matched with modernized counterparts of the same ethnic background, geography, elevation, and climate, whose only difference was their switch to the "nutrition of commerce"—swimming then, as it is now, in white flour, sugar, jams, canned goods, and vegetable oils. In that sense, the groups eating their traditional diets could serve as scientific controls against those who'd abandoned their traditional ways. How did the newly modernized populations compare to their still-isolated brethren? Price summed it up as follows:

> In every instance where individuals of the same racial stocks who had lost this isolation and who had adopted the foods and food habits of our modern civilization were examined, there was an early loss of the high immunity characteristics of the isolated group.[22]

It was a pattern confirmed not just by Price's own observations, but also by medical doctors he encountered throughout his travels—physicians working intimately enough with native populations to grasp their prevalence of disease. In Alaska, for instance, he met Dr. Josef Romig, a somewhat legendary surgeon who'd spent decades treating both primitive and modernized Eskimos and American Indians. Along with graciously introducing Price to the native families he needed for his study, Dr. Romig recounted his observations from many years of hospital work in Anchorage. As Price summarized:

> He stated that in his thirty-six years of contact with these people he had never seen a case of malignant disease [cancer] among the truly primitive Eskimos and Indians, although it frequently occurs when they become modernized. He found similarly that the acute surgical problems requiring operation on internal organs such as the gall bladder, kidney, stomach, and appendix do not tend to occur among the primitive, but are very common problems among the modernized Eskimos and Indians.[23]

What's more, Romig routinely ushered modernized, tuberculosis-stricken Eskimos and Indians back to their traditional diets and lifestyles, which proved to be a remarkably effective protocol: he told Price that "a great majority of the afflicted recover under the primitive type of living and nutrition," helping death rates plummet.[24]

The phenomenon wasn't limited to Alaska, either. In Kenya, a doctor heading the local government hospital assured Price that "Malignancy was ... very rare among the primitives," as were afflictions like appendicitis, gall bladder disease, and ulcers.[25] Similarly, a doctor treating residents of the Torres Strait Islands—another stop on Price's quest—confirmed the absence of cancer among those staying true to their traditional diets:

> Dr. J. R. Nimmo, the government physician in charge of the supervision of this group, told me in his thirteen years with them he had not seen a single case of malignancy, and had seen only one that he had suspected might be malignancy among the entire four thousand native population. He stated that during this same period he had operated several dozen malignancies for the white population, which numbers about three hundred.[26]

Both the beauty and the tragedy of Price's work is that his studies would be all but impossible to re-conduct today. Price caught a snapshot of traditional communities as they teetered on the cusp of modernization—with the following decades quickly swapping their traditional diets, lifestyles, cultures, and legendary physical health with the ways of the West. Unlike retrospectively figuring out the diets of hunter-gatherers from the distant past (a feat involving much guesswork, uncertainty, and perhaps even psychic skills), Price was able to learn about modern "primitive" populations directly from their remaining members. In that sense, Price's work was in a class of its own, and is unlikely to be one-upped by any similar endeavors in the future.

From our modern perspective, where clinical trials and randomized designs typify what we see as "good science," Price's research may seem crude by comparison—an interesting but inconclusive survey of a bygone era. And we've certainly harped on the woes of observational research enough to know that in Price's work, too, cause and effect is impossible to fully tease out. But in some ways, the groups he studied were themselves the products of a rigorous science experiment, one spanning centuries and reaching life-or-death proportions. Sure, those populations didn't have high-tech lab equipment or statistics software or handsome funding from the National Institutes of Health—but they *did* have generation after generation of trial and error. The stakes, for them, were high. Without the luxury of modern medical technology to rescue sick infants and extend the lives of the elderly, these isolated groups had to build the healthiest bodies possible out of the materials their environments provided. And in order to do so, that meant learning the hard way which foods supported health and which foods (or *absence* of foods) led to weakness and disease. Price called the phenomenon "accumulated wisdom," and believed it was a feature utterly lost from modern society:

> In my studies of these several racial stocks I find that it is not accident but accumulated wisdom regarding foods that lies behind their physical excellence and freedom from our modern degenerative processes, and, further, that on various sides of our world the primitive people know many of the things that are essential for life—things that our modern civilizations apparently do not know…. It must be that these various primitive racial stocks have been able through a superior skill in interpreting cause and effect, to determine for themselves what foods in their environment are best for producing human bodies with a maximum of physical fitness and resistance to degeneration.[27]

Not every group Price tracked down showed superb health, nor should we romanticize all native populations as exuding some sort of magic-laced wisdom that steers them toward physical perfection. The groups Price included in his study were only those who had met the criteria for being truly robust. But there were many others that *hadn't* cracked the "good health" code, and due to their environments, suffered from parasitic infestation, starvation, and other serious problems.

Perhaps most pertinent to the theme of this chapter, though, is the fact that Price's groups had dazzlingly diverse menus—while at the same time, prizing certain foods vital for health. Let's take a look at the most exemplary diets that Price encountered. We'll be talking about the common threads afterward, but as you read the following, see if you can identify any overarching patterns.

The Swiss of the Loetschental Valley ate generous amounts of hand-milled rye bread, extraordinarily nutritious dairy products (typically in the form of raw cheese cut as wide as the slice of the bread it was eaten on), meat about once per week, small amounts of butter and raw milk, and an assortment of vegetables—fresh in the summer; stored for winter. Per Price's analyses, the dairy reached nutritional superstardom due to the fast-growing grass carpeting those high alpine valleys: its rich vitamin and mineral content transferred to the milk of the cows lucky enough to nosh on it. In fact, the Swiss so cherished the dairy made in June—when cows ate the luscious summer grass near the snowline—that the people of the Loetschental Valley would hold a type of worship service to pay homage, lighting a wick in a bowl of the first butter of the season and letting it burn in a special sanctuary.[28,29]

The Gaelics in the Outer and Inner Hebrides (an archipelago off the coast of mainland Scotland) consumed a diet rich in oat products—the only grain that thrived in the climate there—with porridge or oat cakes eaten at nearly every meal. Seafood was their other mainstay, with the coastal waters providing ample fish, lobsters, crabs, oysters, and clams. Price noted that an important local dish was cod's head stuffed with oatmeal and chopped cod livers. Although the peat-blanketed land didn't offer much in the way of vegetation, the isolated Gaelics ate vegetables fresh in the summer and stored for winter.[30,31]

The Eskimos of Alaska made liberal use of edible sea life—resulting in a diet high in organ meats and other tissues from various sea animals, along with fish, seal oil (in which salmon was often dipped), seal meat, caribou, and fish eggs. As Price described, the Eskimos "selected certain organs and tissues with great care and wisdom," including the inner layer of skin from a local whale species (which turned out to be one of their few reliable sources of vitamin C). Although plant matter was on the sparser side, the Eskimos collected berries and other vegetation in the summer and saved some for the winter, leading to a small but nutritionally vital supply of cranberries, kelp, water grasses, other water plants, bulbs, ground nuts, and flower blossoms preserved in seal oil.[32,33]

The Native American Indians of the Rocky Mountains consumed wild game—namely moose and caribou—along with bark, tree buds, and some vegetation when it flourished in summertime. Explaining the Native Americans' meat consumption habits, Price noticed something that echoes our "nose to tail" discussion in *Meet Your Meat*:

> I found the Indians putting great emphasis upon the eating of the organs of the animals, including the wall of parts of the digestive tract. *Much of the muscle meat of the animals was fed to the dogs.* ... The skeletal remains [of hunted game animals] are found as piles of finely broken bone chips or splinters that have been cracked up to obtain as much as possible of the bone marrow and nutritive qualities of the bones. (Emphasis mine.)

In other words, the Native Americans prized the very foods—entrails and organs and bones—that we now exile from our diets, and often discarded the muscle meats we've come to favor.[34,35]

The Melanesians and Polynesians on Southern Pacific archipelagos enjoyed diets rich in shellfish and finfish from nearby waters, along with plenty of tubers and tropical fruit. Taro, in particular, was a staple plant whose starchy root and tender leaves (the latter eaten with coconut cream) were both common sights at mealtime. (Some communities would cook the taro root, dry it, pound it to smithereens, and then mix it with water and allow it to ferment for a day or so—

A CAVEAT FOR LOW-CARBERS?

Along with capturing some of our modern diet's missing nutritional pieces (and dumping them back into the puzzle box for us to fiddle with), Price uncovered a potential clue about the long-term impact of very low carbohydrate diets. During his travels, he visited the natives of the far north—whose meat-centered, plant-sparse menu is sometimes cited as evidence that humans can thrive on rock-bottom intakes of carbohydrate. Yet among the inland tribes, an unusual fertility pattern emerged. Pregnancy among the natives depended heavily on their access to the thyroid glands of one of their dietary mainstays, the moose:

> Among the Indians in the moose country near the Arctic Circle a larger percentage of the children were born in June than in any other month. This was accomplished, I was told, by both parents eating liberally of the thyroid glands of the male moose as they came down from the high mountain areas for the mating season, at which time the large protuberances carrying the thyroids under the throat were greatly enlarged.[52]

In other words, the natives appeared to have reduced fertility until a thyroid-gland feast restored it, as indicated by the disproportionate number of babies born nine months later. Incidentally, thyroid hormone is critical for helping your body convert cholesterol into sex hormones, and thus plays a major role in reproductive ability. And carbohydrate intake, in turn, has been linked to both thyroid status and sex hormone levels in humans.[53,54] That suggests these natives' traditional, very-low-carbohydrate diet might not be the best at supporting thyroid health, affecting fertility as a result. Those northerly populations were able to "hack" that dietary insufficiency through a sort of natural medicating: ingesting high amounts of supplementary thyroid hormone from moose.

While low-carb diets haven't unleashed the reign of artery-clogging terror conventional wisdom might predict, and in fact have fared well in most clinical trials, their effect on thyroid status is worth further study.

resulting in a food called *poi,* which you might have seen if you've ever been to Hawaii.)[36,37,38]

The tribes in eastern and central Africa depended largely on what their terrain could handle, but most consumed starchy foods like sweet potatoes, beans, or some grains like corn and millet. Communities near fresh-water lakes and streams feasted on fish, while other tribes frequently hunted wild animals or domesticated goats and cattle to use for meat and dairy. And while the thought may be a gag-reflex trigger for some Westerners, many tribes trapped a creepy, crawly, and incredibly nutritious resource: insects. As Price describes,

> … great swarms of a large winged insect … often accumulated on the shores to a depth of many inches. They were gathered, dried, and preserved to be used in puddings which are highly prized by the natives and are well spoken of by the missionaries. Another insect source of vitamins used frequently by the natives is the ant which is collected from great ant hills that in many districts grow to heights of ten feet or more. … We were told by the missionaries that one of the great luxuries was an ant pie but unfortunately they were not able to supply us with this delicacy. … [Locusts] are gathered in large quantities, to be cooked for immediate use or dried and ground into flour for later use. They provide a rich source of minerals and vitamins.[39,40]

The Australian Aborigines lived on native plants and wild animals—particularly wallabies, kangaroos, rodents, and other small critters. As another example of the nose-to-tail theme, Price noted that the Aborigines ate "all of the edible parts, including the walls of the viscera and internal organs." The communities living by the ocean also made liberal use of seafood.[41,42]

The Maori of New Zealand were yet another seafood-loving population, mining the ocean for its bounty—favoring certain species of shellfish, in particular, due to their "unique nutritive value." Inland, the Maori captured fatty muttonbirds just before they fled the nest, and made use of the region's abundant fruits and vegetables, including large quantities of fern root. In school, rather than bringing food from home, Maori children would make a beeline for the beach as soon as their lunch break arrived—only to set up bonfires, strip down, plunge into the sea, and wrangle giant lobsters back to the shore. "The lobsters were promptly roasted on the coals and devoured with great relish," Price described. (Compare that feast with the goldfish crackers and Capri Suns filling kids' lunch boxes today.[43,44])

The Malay tribes on islands north of Australia were lucky enough to live in a hotbed of marine life, near waters harboring some of the largest shellfish and richest pearl fisheries in the world—giving them an enormous supply of ocean edibles. (The shellfish, in fact, were so big that Price commonly saw their shells used as full-sized washtubs.) A large marine mammal called dugong, also known as a sea cow, was another prized food source. Describing the area's abundance of seafood, Price wrote:

> The fish in the water at times form such a dense mass that they can be scooped into the boats directly from the sea. Fishermen wading out in the surf and throwing their spears into the schools of fish usually impale one or several.

In addition, the island tribes ate a variety of plant roots, greens, and fruit—the latter growing abundantly in the tropical climate.[45]

The Indians of the Andean Highlands ate an abundance of potatoes, llama meat, and guinea pigs—which, hardy little creatures that they were, flourished in colonies in the high-altitude terrain and were often used in stews. The Andean Indians also regularly consumed dried fish eggs, which they told Price was necessary for maintaining the fertility of their women. Likewise, they ate an abundance of mineral-rich kelp to avoid getting "big necks" like the Europeans (no doubt referring to goiter caused by iodine deficiency).[46,47]

Quite a whirlwind, right? For starters, we can see that no particular level of carbohydrate or fat intake, ratio of plant foods to animal foods, or any other of today's hotly debated diet topics seemed to matter much in terms of maintaining healthy communities. Nor did a single food emerge as essential across all cultures.

Some groups ate grains, though generally with more foresight than we eat ours—including a preparation of soaking, sprouting, or fermenting to remove antinutrients like phytates. Some groups ate dairy, valuing the high-vitamin butterfat during its seasonal peaks. Some groups were nearly pescetarian, eating little in the way of flesh beyond fish. Some groups had to make do with low levels of edible plants growing in their harsh environments. Yet in every instance Price recorded, bone formation reached perfection, degenerative disease seemed absent, and teeth were nearly immune to decay. How do we make sense of it all?

It turns out these diverse diets do have some things in common: most notably, their nutrient density. Describing the health-promoting versus health-depleting diets he encountered in his travels, Price wrote that across the board, the cuisines associated with "very high immunity to dental caries and freedom from other degenerative processes" contained at least four times the level of vitamins and minerals recommended by American nutritionists.

And among those nutrients, the fat-soluble vitamins—A, D, E, and K—emerged as the most critical, as well as the most notably absent from modernized menus. (If you'll recall from *Herbivore's Dilemma,* these nutrients are particularly vital for bone formation, tooth development, cell division, gene expression, reproduction, immunity, vision, and other fun things.)

Likewise, none of those health-promoting diets were strictly vegan. Price, in fact, had been actively searching for societies living on plant matter alone—only to acknowledge at the end of his travels, "I have not found a single group of primitive racial stock which was building and maintaining excellent bodies by living entirely on plant foods." Continuing, he wrote,

> I have found in many parts of the world most devout representatives of modern ethical systems advocating the restriction of foods to the vegetable products. In every instance where the groups involved had been long under this teaching, I found evidence of degeneration in the form of dental caries, and in the new generation in the form of abnormal dental arches to an extent very much higher than in the primitive groups who were not under this influence.[48]

A less obvious thread of dietary unity was in the particular foods each group held in high regard: the summertime butter for the Swiss, the cod liver for the Gaelic, the organ meats and whale skin for the Eskimos, the fish eggs for the Andean Indians, and so on. In every instance, the prized foods were a rich source—sometimes the only source—of fat-soluble vitamins, and the isolated groups independently concluded they were imperative for health.

Going back to Price's concept of "accumulated wisdom," it seems those endless generations of trial and error had united groups across the globe in at least one shared belief: the importance of those fat-soluble-vitamin rich foods. In addition, the diets most closely linked with stellar dental health and freedom from degenerative disease were also united in what they *didn't* include—namely, heavily processed grains, sugars, and vegetable oils. That's beautifully consistent with the same areas of overlap we saw when comparing Paleolithic, plant-based, and Mediterranean diets.

Takeaway Points

Although Price's work was fairly spectacular as far as observational studies go, we still run into that little conundrum of *correlation doesn't imply causation*, and the burning questions: Which parts of each traditional diet truly bestowed health? Were the prized items as beneficial as each group believed, or just imbued with the relics of superstition? How much of the primitive populations' health was owed to non-dietary factors such as fresh air and physical activity?

Although we can make educated guesses on those matters, we can't know with the same confidence we'd get from a tightly controlled clinical trial. And in that sense, we should acknowledge that any deductions we make from Price's work might be incomplete or inconclusive. However, even with the most cautious and restrained interpretation of his findings, we *can* say the following with some certainty:

1. It is possible for human beings to be in fabulous health—with hardy bodies, strong immunity to both chronic and infectious disease, and, of course, a great set of pearly whites without retainers and bleaching kits. In other words, our modern disease-stricken state doesn't have to be the norm, and neither do endless fillings and root canals.

VEGGIE TALES

Generally speaking, the "highly prized" foods of each community Price investigated were of animal origin, with no community living on a plant-only diet. That doesn't imply the optimal diet for mankind is necessarily meat based; it often took only small quantities of those items to work their purported magic, after all. Nor does it mean a diet must be high in fat in order to be beneficial: many of the healthy tribes ate starch-based diets, with fatty, nutrient-dense animal foods used at more supplementary levels. But the consistency of certain animal foods linking with fertility and optimal development *does* raise the question of whether a plant-only diet can bring vitality across the span of generations. Is our understanding of nutrition advanced enough to identify, isolate, and fill in every missing nutritional gap that comes when animal foods are off the table? Will the successes we've seen with vegan (or near-vegan) diets in clinical settings continue over the course of a lifetime, supporting robust offspring as well? These are currently unknowns.

2. The populations Price studied were able to reach—and maintain—that state of stellar health on their traditional diets, generation after generation. Though we don't know for sure what aspect of those diets contributed to such great results, we do know that nothing they ate stood in the way.

3. The diversity of the traditional diets shows there's no single "optimum" for all humans; rather, it seems some important nutritional bases need to be covered, particularly in the form of fat-soluble vitamins that have been on the decline in Westernized nations. Grains don't appear to be universally necessary for producing health; ditto for both dairy and meat from land animals, which were sparse or absent in many coastal regions, as long as fat-soluble vitamins make their way into the diet through another reliable avenue.

4. None of the groups ate anything resembling the USDA's refined-grain-permissive, vegetable-oil-filled, lowfat-dairy-pushing food pyramid. If anything, the traditional diets universally prized foods that would get shelved on the pyramid's tip due to their high cholesterol or saturated fat content.

(Price did note that the seafood-eating cultures were particularly remarkable in terms of physical build and health, writing, "I have been impressed with the superior quality of the human stock developed by Nature wherever a liberal source of sea foods existed."[49])

Ultimately, what Price discovered—and what's often left out of today's nutritional philosophizing—is that health declines not just with the introduction of certain foods, but with the *loss* of certain foods. Even the most health-conscious among us often focuses more on avoiding the well-known "bad guys" (say, sugar and soda and the donuts in the break room), without giving equal thought to the vital foods that should be consumed. The items that *do* gain a social rep for being beneficial tend to earn their *superfood* status through heavy marketing rather than good science—think soy products, goji berries, acai, noni juice, and other dietary darlings hyped to the moon and back. The foods that may be the biggest treasure trove for human health, if Price's findings are any indication, are ones that have been virtually eradicated due to cultural stigmas and fearmongering: organ meats and offal, high-cholesterol fish eggs and shellfish, insects, bones and bone marrow, and high-fat dairy from cows eating lush grass.

In that sense, our modern diet poses a double whammy of woe. We're feasting on heavily processed, new-to-the-human-body foods that may inherently be damaging while neglecting the best health-building items out there.

Of course, Price's work delivered another message as well. **You're not just what you eat: you are what your mom ate. And what your grandmother ate. And what your food eats, given how soil and pasturage quality influenced the nutritional status of native diets.** Price's saga, in one sense, should expand our view of nutrition to encompass more than our fork's journey from the plate to the mouth.

Context Is Everything

Ultimately, Price's work captures the message behind this chapter—and in some sense, behind this book at large—that chasing a single ideal diet is the wrong way to approach health. While we frantically hop from one eating plan to the next, searching for physical perfection by eating the right amount of carbs or fat or synthetic vitamins or grapefruit slices, we miss the bigger picture—and with it, the opportunity to truly nourish our bodies.

Of course, there's one major problem with applying work like Price's to our own lives: *context.* These days, most of us aren't born into families who've been eating stellar diets for generation after generation, or living in pristine environments with fresh air and mineral-rich soil, or avoiding stress and sleep deprivation and those other thorns in the side of modern living. Many of us were born already saddled with the bad food karma of our forbearers, so to speak, thanks to parents and grandparents eating the white flour and refined sugar and industrialized vegetable oils lauded in days past.

Or maybe we were doing all right when we were evicted from the womb, but environmental abuses—such as a poor diet, gut-flora-obliterating antibiotics, and other conditions—altered our bodies in a way where simply mimicking the diet of a traditional population won't be enough to restore our health. It may be that the nutritional playing field changes once we've hit a certain level of "brokenness." Or that diets optimal for *maintaining* health fall short once a disease is already seeded. It could be that healing from generations of poor health requires a specialized menu—hence the apparently therapeutic effects of grain-free diets (despite the existence of healthy grain-eating populations in the past), or low-carbohydrate diets (despite the existence of healthy high-carbohydrate-eating populations in the past), or dairy-free diets (despite the existence of healthy dairy-eating populations in the past), and so on.

This is where we'll interrupt our regularly scheduled programming for a special announcement from *individual variation.*

Individuality:
You're More Than a Peer-Reviewed Statistic

I'm sure this sounds like a self-esteem building exercise from third grade—*You are an individual! You are a special snowflake!*—but bear with me. The concept of individuality in nutritional needs isn't just some gimmick to sell you expensive supplements and hook you onto a slapdash, scientifically tenuous diet based on your blood type or eye color or favorite David Bowie song. It's simply a genetic reality. And it goes a long way to help reconcile how one of your friends could shed eighty pounds following Atkins while another claims they've never been slimmer or more energetic since going lowfat vegan.

In previous chapters, we've already explored some of the ways your body can be special in its reaction to certain foods or diets. Here's a recap of some, as well as a few newbies thrown in for good measure.

Amylase individuality. Depending on how much amylase you produce in your saliva, you may fare beautifully on high-starch diets, or crash and burn like the Hindenburg. (See page 205.)

ApoE individuality. The ApoE alleles you carry play a role in lipid metabolism and may influence how you respond to dietary cholesterol and saturated fat—an important caution if you're embarking on a high-fat diet. Other apolipoproteins, including A-I, A-IV, and B, may also play a role in lipid response to diet.[50] (See page 133.)

Carotene-to-retinol conversion individuality. Topnotch converters stand a better chance at doing well on vegetarian or vegan diets; poor converters are likely to experience problems related to vitamin A, no matter how many carrots they mow down. (See page 203.)

Metabolic individuality. Current research suggests that folks with insulin resistance respond better to low-carbohydrate diets than to lowfat diets.[51] (See pages 114-133.)

Lactose tolerance (or intolerance) individuality. If you've lost the ability to produce the lactase enzyme, which works its magic on the milk sugar lactose, then most dairy won't be your dietary friend.

Gut flora individuality. The critters in your gut—influenced by everything from antibiotic usage to stress to the microbes you picked up whooshing out of your mom's birth canal—can influence your response to different foods and diet patterns.

The list goes on. Depending on how deep you want to dive in (and how large of a nerd badge you're willing to tote around), you can even analyze your own genetic background through companies like 23andMe.com, which will grant you a fascinating peephole into, well, you.

And one more thing: we ought not assume diets that help *reverse* chronic conditions would also be necessary to help prevent them in the first place. A healthy leg doesn't need to wear a cast, but a broken one might, until it heals. The same goes with many of the diets out there. Some of us might need short-term therapeutic menus to expedite the healing process and restore our body's equilibrium. But our goal should be to regain the ability to handle a broad spectrum of healthful foods, not lock ourselves into a restrictive program for life. For that reason, it's important not to immediately pledge eternal allegiance to a diet that helped pry you out of a medical jam, just because it worked fabulously for a few months or a year. Often an "emergency diet" is different than a maintenance diet.

Take-Home Kit

Considering we've just painstakingly explored the evidence that no single diet is optimal for all people, I'm not letting you depart with a specific meal plan or recipe guide to guarantee you Rock Star Health. There *are* a few clear themes that emerge when we synthesize all the findings we've looked at so far, and those are jewels you should pluck out of this book, place in your pocket, and carry with you for as long as they serve you. Here are the biggies.

Eliminate or drastically reduce your intake of refined grains, refined sugar, and high-omega-6 vegetable oils. No healthy human population has thrived on these items, and the bulk of the evidence points toward their harm.

Secure a source of those precious fat-soluble vitamins—whether from shellfish, fish eggs, high-quality dairy, bone marrow, organ meats like liver, or cod liver oil. Even small amounts can go a long way. (If you're a committed vegan, this part is trickier: optimize your chance of nutrient-conversion success by following the tips outlined in *Herbivore's Dilemma,* and consider adding bivalves to your diet, which aren't sentient.)

Stock your diet with nutrient-dense items from both the plant kingdom and the animal kingdom—a spectrum including seaweeds, wild greens, fermented vegetables, berries, mushrooms, and the animal foods listed above.

When choosing animal foods, limit muscle meat and favor "nose to tail" eating.

Respect your genetics. If you react to high-fat, low-carbohydrate diets with skyrocketing LDL and other worsening blood markers, that way of eating may not be right for you. Same goes if you're a sparse amylase producer and find yourself on a ravenous energy roller-coaster while attempting a high-starch diet.

Acknowledge that health is about a lot more than what you put in your mouth, and treat yourself kindly in all areas of life—which means getting enough sleep, exercising, minimizing stress, maintaining strong social connections, getting fresh air and sunshine, and taking care of your psychological and emotional well-being.

Above all else, stay anchored in your own truth rather than falling under the spell of groupthink. Just as we shouldn't outsource our thinking to gurus and federal branches that don't always have our best interest at heart, we shouldn't outsource the interpretation of our experiences to minds other than our own.

And Remember: You Are Not a Jar

While labels can be handy for zippy-quick descriptions of what you eat—serving as great elevator pitches about your dietary choices or helping you gain acceptance into local potlucks where you won't feel like a freak of nature—they can also become a psychological trap that prevents you from following your body's instincts.

If you choose to put a label on your diet, make sure it doesn't undergo a sneaky "mission creep" into the realm of your self-identity. Your current food choices may be low-carb, or lowfat, or plant-based, or any other number of descriptors—but *you* are not low-carb; *you* are not lowfat; *you* are not plant-based. You're a human being trying to make choices that best serve you and your specific goals at this point in time. You are not defined by the foods you eat. You are not a slave to an ideology. Make your diet work for you; don't work for your diet.

Afterword

IN THE FINAL SUN-DAPPLED DAYS of writing this book—on one of my many brainstorming, thought-simmering, Greek-muse-summoning walks around Northeast Portland—I found myself standing in front of a breathtaking sight: figs. They were stacked in a kingdom of green plastic pints alongside an equally beautiful sign: "ON SALE."

This is not an uncommon occurrence. Come late summer, figs are to me what tartan is to a Scot, shoes to a shopaholic, Johnny Depp to a Tim Burton film. My fig standards are high: buying them is an elaborate ritual of squeezing, inspecting, prodding, rearranging, and swapping until I've groped every fruit within reach and traded the plumpest into a single pint (usually earning some employee stink-eyes in the process). If I carried anything with me from my raw vegan stint, it's fruit snobbery.

But on this particular day, fig-buying was more about giving my hands something to busy themselves with while my brain mulled the end of a tome I spent two-and-a-half years of my life writing. And as I absently squeezed each piece of fruit, my attention suddenly turned to an elderly woman standing next to me, who had been observing my elaborate routine. For just how long, I'm not sure. But I half expected a lecture about manhandling the store's bounty.

Instead, she offered me a smile.

"We used to pick these off the trees on our way home from school when I was growing up," the woman said wistfully. "They grew every-where, these purple ones. So good. We hardly ever paid for food back then."

She looked at me with a classic movie-moment eye sparkle—time weathering her face but sparing, it seemed, the blue jewel of her irises. It's as if she knew she'd captured the message resting at the core of this book.

That woman's childhood existed in an era long-since bulldozed into folklore. A time buried deep enough in memory for her to look back on it with a sense of permanent loss. (Granted, I sometimes pick figs on my way home, too, but those ventures are usually cut short when someone yells at me to get off their lawn.)

And that's the point: like most people, my hands have little to do with the growth or harvesting of the foods I so cherish.

It's a clear but tragic symptom of the direction our nation, and more broadly our world, is heading. Over the years, we've become increasingly disconnected from the food we eat—the way it's produced, the journey it takes from farm to fork, the source of our beliefs about its goodness or badness, its place in the meandering history of humankind. We hunt and gather in the store, seduced by alluring packaging and clever marketing. We absorb whatever dietary advice we grew up with and often spend a lifetime never questioning it. Just as that woman's childhood fig-picking is now a nostalgia-laced relic, our physical and intellectual drift from our food suggests a future where the "good ol' days" will be the ones we're living *now.*

No doubt, this is a fascinating, pivotal, and somewhat terrifying time to be on planet earth—an era of unprecedented opportunities, global connectedness, and the entire universe accessible with a quick whirr of the Google machine. But as much as we're living big, we're also living sick. The mistakes of our past have reached a critical mass. Our medical technology, with all its bells and whistles, may soon fail to keep pace with the graves we're digging with the shovels of self-destructive lifestyles and diet. The current generation may, for the first time in memory, die younger than the one that came before it. Rates of "new" diseases and autoimmune conditions are crippling us like never before. Around the globe, governments are wrapping their already-long arms around wider chunks of nutritional territory, issuing not only public policies and dietary guides, but—as seen in Denmark's short-lived "fat tax"—deterring sales of items conventional wisdom has deemed unhealthy. Playing with our food has taken on new meaning, with biotechnology giant Monsanto steering the future of our crops and livestock toward genetic modification, often with questionable safety testing. The changes are rapid and escalating by the day.

We need a new direction, and we need it soon. Instead of death by food pyramid, we can have *life* by educated freedom—a freedom in which we're released from the rules of the federal government, the dogma of the fad diet du jour, the smooth words of a health guru, the marionetting of powerful industries, the misinterpretation of science, and the mass confusion that keeps us incapacitated. As we demolish the walls of the pyramids, plates, and other shapes that ultimately lock us inside a dietary dictatorship, we're left with a horizon-wide landscape to explore—and with it, the opportunity to pursue what works for us and guiltlessly leave behind what doesn't.

But there's just one catch. In order to reach that point of liberation, we can't keep doing what we've been doing—or else we'll keep getting what we've been getting. Einstein's specialty wasn't exactly diet, but when he sagely said, "You can't solve a problem with the same mind that created it," he might as well have been talking about nutrition. Neither sweeping public policies nor trendy diets demanding your full allegiance have bred a nation of healthy humans.

It's one thing to learn how our food recommendations went awry; it's another beast entirely to actually do something about it. If knowledge is power, then action is the electrical circuitry that pours it toward something worthwhile. This is not the time to wait for change. It's a time to consciously make it happen. As a consumer—one who, if you've made it this far into the book without shoving it under a wobbly chair leg, is clearly interested in the state of our health and the politics in which it's ensnared—you're in a unique position to help shift the tides. You're a vital drop in a sea of potential change. You're equipped with spending power, voting power, intellectual power. It's time to use it.

We're locked in a global food fight that's as personal as it is political—one we as consumers stand no chance at winning unless we stand up and demand, through the votes of our dollars and ballots and words, the freedom of choice. The burden is on our own shoulders to stay educated, informed, shrewd, critical, proactive, and unyielding in the face of the Goliaths that loom before us.

So stand up and sling your stone. Or fig, if there's one within reach.

Notes

1. Pyramid is the New Paradigm

1. Carole Sugarman and Malcom Gladwell, "U.S. Drops New Food Chart: Meat, dairy groups pressure the Agriculture Department," *Washington Post,* April 27, 1991.
2. "A Pyramid Topples at the USDA," *Consumer Reports,* (October 1991): 663-6.
3. Sugarman and Gladwell, "U.S. Drops New Food Chart: Meat, dairy groups pressure the Agriculture Department."
4. Marian Burros, "Eating Well; Rethink 4 Food Groups, Doctors Tell U.S.," *New York Times,* April 10, 1991.
5. James S. Todd, "Keep Meat and Dairy Products in Diet," *New York Times,* May 8, 1991.
6. Marion Nestle, "Dietary Advice for the 1990s: The Political History of the Food Guide Pyramid," *Caduceus: A Humanities Journal for Medicine and the Health Sciences* 9, no. 3 (1993): 131-51.
7. "Forget USDA, Dump Food Wheel," *Sun Sentinel,* May 1, 1991.
8. Sugarman and Gladwell, "U.S. Drops New Food Chart: Meat, dairy groups pressure the Agriculture Department."
9. Otis Pike, "USDA Casts Doubt on Its Integrity," *Chicago Sun-Times,* May 15, 1991.
10. Marion Nestle, *Food Politics* (Berkley and Los Angeles: University of California Press, 2012), 51.
11. Ibid.
12. "'Pyramid' Points to Healthy Diet," *Chicago Tribune,* April 29, 1992.
13. Ibid.
14. Robin Branch, "Where's the Beef With New Diet Plan?" *Sun Sentinel,* May 3, 1992.
15. Nestle, "Dietary Advice for the 1990s: The Political History of the Food Guide Pyramid."

16. Jeff Nesmith, "Government Unveils Long-Delayed Food Pyramid," *The News Journal*, April 29, 1992.

17. Marian Burros, "U.S. Reorganizes Nutrition Advice," *New York Times*, April 28, 1992.

18. "A Pyramid-Sized Fizzle," *The Shopper Report*, June 1, 1992.

19. Barbara Bell Matuszewski, "The Low-Fat Lowdown: A State of the Union Report on Americans' Love-Hate Affair With Fat," *Restaurants and Institutions*, August 1, 1996.

20. Candy Sagon, "A Hard Pyramid to Swallow? You Bet it Is—And I have a Kitchen Full of Bread and Pasta to Prove it," *Washington Post*, April 28, 1993.

21. Edward N. Siguel and Robert H. Lerman, "Role of Essential Fatty Acids: Dangers in the U.S. Department of Agriculture Dietary Recommendations ("Pyramid") and in Low-Fat Diets," *American Journal of Clinical Nutrition* 60, no. 6 (1994): 973-4.

22. Walter Willet, "The Dietary Pyramid: Does the Foundation Need Repair?" *American Journal of Clinical Nutrition* 68, no. 2 (1998): 218-9.

23. Patricia Bertron, Neal Barnard, and Milton Mills, "Racial Bias in Federal Nutrition Policy, Part I: The Public Health Implications of Variations in Lactase Persistence," *Journal of the National Medical Association* 91, no. 3 (1999): 151-7.

24. Laura F. Thomas, "Food Guide Pyramid Stimulates Debate," *Journal of the American Dietetic Association* 95, no. 3 (1995): 297.

25. Mary Abbott Hess, "Food Guide Pyramid Stimulates Debate," *Journal of the American Dietetic Association* 95, no. 3 (1995): 297.

26. "School Meals Initiative Summary," *California Department of Education*, accessed August 14, 2012, http://web.archive.org/web/20100316090236/http://www.cde.ca.gov/ls/nu/he/smismmary.asp.

27. Carole A. Davis, Patricia Britten, and Esther Myers, "Past, Present, and Future of the Food Guide Pyramid," *Journal of the American Dietetic Association* 101, no. 8 (2001): 881-5.

28. "Prices are Rising and Palme is Silent," *SR Memories*, accessed January 14, 2013, http://sverigesradio.se/sida/artikel.aspx?programid=1602&artikel=775692.

29. "The Test Kitchen Became Test Kitchens," *Cooperative Chronicle*, last modified October 3, 2008, http://www.mersmak.kf.se/Toppmeny-startsida-/KFBibliotek/Kooperativ-kronika-startsida/Sok/KF-Kronika---Visa-artikel/?articleid=641.

30. Ibid.

2. Design by Committee

1. Luise Light, *What to Eat* (New York: McGraw Hill, 2006), 13.
2. Ibid., 15.
3. Ibid., 16.
4. Luise Light, "A Fatally Flawed Food Guide," *Conscious Choice*, last modified November 2004, http://web.archive.org/web/20090207074229/http://consciouschoice.com/2004/cc1711/wh_lead1711.html.
5. "The Food Guide Pyramid," United States Department of Agriculture, accessed October 7, 2013, http://www.cnpp.usda.gov/Publications/MyPyramid/OriginalFoodGuidePyramids/FGP/FGPPamphlet.pdf.
6. Light, *What to Eat*, 18.
7. "Food and Agriculture Act of 1977: Public Law 95-113, sec. 1502(a), 91 Stat. 1021, 7 U.S.C. 2201," National Institutes of Health, September 29, 1997, http://history.nih.gov/research/downloads/PL95-113.pdf.
8. Sander L. Gilman, *Fat: A Cultural History of Obesity* (Cambridge: Polity Press, 2008), 16.
9. Carole Davis and Etta Saltos, "Dietary Recommendations and How They Have Changed Over Time," in *America's Eating Habits: Changes and Consequences,* ed. Elizabeth Frazao (Washington, DC: Economic Research Service, 1999), 33-50.
10. Caroline L. Hunt, "Food For Young Children," *United States Department of Agriculture Farmers' Bulletin,* no. 717, March 4, 1916, http://openlibrary.org/books/OL24364099M/Food_for_young_children.
11. Davis and Saltos, "Dietary Recommendations and How They Have Changed Over Time."

3. Amber Waves of Shame

1. "Video: Making America Stronger: U.S. Food Stamp Program," *Center on Budget and Policy Priorities,* March 8, 2007, http://www.cbpp.org/cms/index.cfm?fa=view&id=1274.

2. Richard Goldstein, "Earl L. Butz, Secretary Felled by Racial Remark, Is Dead at 98," *New York Times,* February 4, 2008, http://www.nytimes.com/2008/02/04/washington/04butz.html?_r=0.

3. "Food Conference: Let Them Eat Words?" *Science News* 1, no. 18 (1974): 278.

4. "'Meet the Press' Transcript for July 15, 2007," NBC News, aired July 15, 2007, transcript, http://www.nbcnews.com/id/19694666/page/7/.

5. Michael Pollan, *Omnivore's Dilemma* (New York: Penguin Press, 2006), 52.

6. Michael Leahy, "What Might Have Been," *Washington Post,* February 20, 2005.

7. Joe McGinniss, "Second Thoughts of George McGovern," *New York Times,* May 6, 1973, http://select.nytimes.com/gst/abstract.html?res=F20B13FD3954137A93C4A9178ED85F478785F9.

8. "Biography: Nathan Pritikin, Founder," Pritikin Longevity Center and Spa, accessed February 20, 2013, www.pritikin.com/home-the-basics/about-pritikin/press-room/item/biography-nathan-pritikin-founder.html.

9. Ibid.

10. Joe D. Goldstrich, personal phone interview, February 8, 2013.

11. "McGovern Lauds Pritikin," *Milwaukee Sentinel,* March 1, 1985.

12. Darrell Sifford, "A Dozen Years Later, McGovern Defends Diet Recommendations," *Spokane Chronicle,* March 4, 1986.

13. Curtis Rist, "McGovern Tastefully Moderate," *Inquirer,* February 6, 1988.

14. Sifford, "A Dozen Years Later, McGovern Defends Diet Recommendations."

15. Ibid.

16. Eugenia Killoran, "The Remarkable Friendship of Senator George McGovern and Nathan Pritikin," Pritikin Longevity Center and Spa, accessed February 20, 2013, http://www.pritikin.com/success-stories/194-myblog/1706.html.

17. William J. Broad, "NIH Deals Gingerly with Diet-Disease Link," *Science* 204, no. 4398 (1979): 1175-8.

18. Gary Taubes, personal email correspondence, February 6, 2013.

19. Broad, "NIH Deals Gingerly with Diet-Disease Link."

20. George McGovern, "Statement of Senator George McGovern on the Publication of Dietary Goals for the United States," in *Dietary Goals for the United States* (Washington, D.C.: U.S. Government Printing Office, 1977).

21. Nick Mottern, personal phone interview, July 1, 2013.

22. Mark Hegsted, interview by Henry Blackburn, "Washington: Dietary Guidelines," accessed January 24, 2013, http://www.foodpolitics.com/wp-content/uploads/Hegsted.pdf.

23. Ethel Nelson, "Health and Religion," *Ministry Magazine,* March 1978, https://www.ministrymagazine.org/archive/1978/03/health-and-religion.

24. Hegsted, "Washington: Dietary Guidelines."

25. Ibid.

26. Mark Hegsted, "U.S. Dietary Goals," *Family Economics Review* ARS-NE 36, Winter-Spring 1978.

27. Alfred Harper, "Dietary Goals: A Skeptical View," *American Journal of Clinical Nutrition* 31, no. 2 (1978): 310-21.

28. William J. Broad, "Jump in Funding Feeds Research on Nutrition," *Science* 204, no. 4397 (1979): 1060-4.

29. Ibid.

30. Gilbert A. Leveille, "Establishing and Implementing Dietary Goals," *Family Economics Review* 36 (1978): 7-11.

31. Broad, "NIH Deals Gingerly with Diet-Disease Link."

32. Edward H. Ahrens, "Introduction," *American Journal of Clinical Nutrition* 32, no. 12 (1979): 2627-31.

33. Charles J. Glueck, "Appraisal of Dietary Fat as a Causative Factor in Atherogenesis," *American Journal of Clinical Nutrition* 32, no. 12 (1979): 2637-43.

34. Broad, "NIH Deals Gingerly with Diet-Disease Link."

35. Sifford, "A Dozen Years Later, McGovern Defends Diet Recommendations."

36. Michael Greger, "The McGovern Report," *NutritionFacts.org,* YouTube Video, April 12, 2013, http://nutritionfacts.org/video/the-mcgovern-report/.

37. Nick Mottern, personal phone interview, July 1, 2013.
38. Sifford, "A Dozen Years Later, McGovern Defends Diet Recommendations."
39. Broad, "Jump in Funding Feeds Research on Nutrition."
40. Broad, "NIH Deals Gingerly with Diet-Disease Link."
41. "Dietary Guidelines for Americans," *Department of Health and Human Services and the U.S. Department of Agriculture,* February 1980, http://www.health.gov/dietaryguidelines/1980thin.pdf.
42. Goldstein, "Earl L. Butz, Secretary Felled by Racial Remark, Is Dead at 98."
43. Michael Carlson, "Obituary: Earl Butz," *Guardian,* February 3, 2008.
44. "Butz Praises Hike in Exports," *Miami News,* October 8, 1973.
45. Carlson, "Obituary: Earl Butz."
46. Barbara Sibbald, "Sugar Industry Sour on WHO Report," *Canadian Medical Association Journal* 168, no. 12 (2003): 1585.

4. Evaluating the Experts

1. "False Food Fads Number 39: Physician Gives List of Harmful Diet Doctrines That Have Become Popular," *Washington Post,* April 10, 1910.
2. Errol Morris, "The Anosognosic's Dilemma: Something's Wrong But You'll Never Know What It Is (Part I)," *New York Times,* June 20, 2010.
3. Ibid.
4. Charles Darwin, *The Descent of Man* (London: John Murray, 1871), 4.
5. "Course Requirements in Years I and II," Harvard Medical School, accessed March 12, 2013, http://hms.harvard.edu/content/course-and-examination-requirements-md-degree.
6. Kelly M. Adams, Martin Kohlmeier, and Steven H. Zeisel, "Status of Nutrition Education in Medical Schools," *American Journal of Clinical Nutrition* 83, no. 4 (2006): 941S-4S.
7. Ibid.
8. Eric G. Campbell et al., "A National Survey of Physician-Industry Relationships," *New England Journal of Medicine* 356, no. 17 (2007): 1742-50.

9. Brian Hodges, "Interactions With the Pharmaceutical Industry: Experiences and Attitudes of Psychiatry Residents, Interns and Clerks," *Canadian Medical Association Journal* 153, no. 5 (1995): 553-9.

10. "Opinion 8.061—Gifts to Physicians From Industry," *Journal of the American Medical Association,* accessed January 14, 2013, http://www.ama-assn.org/ama/pub/physician-resources/medical-ethics/code-medical-ethics/opinion8061.page.

11. Susan L. Coyle, "Physician-Industry Relations. Part 1: Individual Physicians," *Annals of Internal Medicine* 136, no. 5 (2002): 396-402.

12. Ben Goldacre, "Dr. Gillian McKeith (PhD) Continued," *Guardian,* September 29, 2004, http://www.guardian.co.uk/science/2004/sep/30/badscience.research.

13. Ellie McGrath, "Education: Sending Degrees to the Dogs," *Time,* April 2, 1984, http://www.time.com/time/magazine/article/0,9171,954229-1,00.html.

14. "The Chaser's War on Everything," *Australian Broadcasting Corporation,* Season 2, Episode 10, May 30, 2007.

15. "Who Are the Academy's Corporate Sponsors?" Academy of Nutrition and Dietetics, accessed July 3, 2013, http://www.eatright.org/corporatesponsors.

16. "Why Become an Academy Sponsor?" Academy of Nutrition and Dietetics, accessed July 3, 2013, http://www.eatright.org/HealthProfessionals/content.aspx?id=10665.

17. "Obesity Myths," accessed June 28, 2013, http://www.obesity-myths.com/.

18. "Trans Fat: Fact and Fiction," The Center For Consumer Freedom, September 28, 2006, http://www.consumerfreedom.com/2006/09/3140-trans-fat-fact-and-fiction/.

19. "Sweet Scam," accessed April 3, 2013, http://www.sweetscam.com/.

20. "Additional Links," The Center for Consumer Freedom, accessed April 3, 2013, http://www.consumerfreedom.com/.

5. The Hitchhiker's Guide to Nutritional Research

1. Richard Horton, "Genetically Modified Food: Consternation, Confusion, and Crack-Up," *Medical Journal of Australia* 172, no. 4 (2000): 148-9.

2. Drummond Rennie et al., "Fifth International Congress on Peer Review and Biomedical Publication," *Journal of the American Medical Association* 289, no. 11 (2003): 1438.

3. "Western Diet for Rodents," *TestDiet,* last modified September 4, 2013, http://www.testdiet.com/cs/groups/lolweb/@testdiet/documents/web_content/mdrf/mdi2/~edisp/ducm04_026663.pdf.

4. Craig H. Warden and Janis S. Fisler, "Comparisons of Diets Used in Animal Models of High Fat Feeding," *Cell Metabolism* 7, no. 4 (2008): 277.

6. Reopening the Case Against Saturated Fat

1. Igor E. Konstantinov, Nicolai Mejevoi, and Nikolai M. Anichkov, "Nikolai N. Anichkov and His Theory of Atherosclerosis," *Texas Heart Institute Journal* 33, no. 4 (2006): 417-23.

2. Daniel Steinberg, *The Cholesterol Wars: The Skeptics vs. the Preponderance of Evidence* (San Diego: Academic Press, 2007), 23.

3. Ibid, 22.

4. Nikolai Anitschkow and S. Chalatow, trans. Mary Z. Pelias, "On Experimental Cholesterolin Steatosis and Its Significance in the Origin of Some Pathological Processes," *Arteriosclerosis* 3, no. 2 (1983): 178-82.

5. Fred Kern, "Normal Cholesterol in an 88-Year-Old Man Who Eats 25 Eggs a Day—Mechanisms of Adaptation," *New England Journal of Medicine* 324, no. 13 (1991): 896-9.

7. Ancel Keys and the Diet-Heart Hypothesis

1. William Hoffman, "Meet Monsieur Cholesterol, *University of Minnesota Update,* 1979, http://mbbnet.umn.edu/hoff/hoff_ak.html.

2. Hardy Green, "How K-Rations Fed Soldiers, Saved Businesses," *San Antonio Express-News*, March 4, 2013, http://www.mysanantonio.com/opinion/commentary/article/How-K-rations-fed-soldiers-saved-businesses-4327409.php.

3. "Battles of Belief in World War II: A Duty to Starve," American RadioWorks, accessed March 13, 2013, http://americanradioworks.publicradio.org/features/wwii/a1.html.

4. "Battles of Belief in World War II: A Duty to Starve."

5. Myrna Oliver, "Ancel Keys, 100; Diet Researcher Developed K-Rations for Troops," *Los Angeles Times,* November 25, 2004, http://articles.latimes.com/2004/nov/25/local/me-keys25.

6. Ibid.

7. Ancel Keys, "Atherosclerosis: a Problem in Newer Public Health" (paper presented at the symposium on Recent Advances In Therapy at Mt. Sinai Hospital, New York City, January 7, 1953).

8. Henry Blackburn, "Famous Polemics on Diet-Heart Theory," *Preventing Heart Attack and Stroke: A History of Cardiovascular Disease Epidemiology,* University of Minnesota, http://www.epi. umn.edu/cvdepi/essay.asp?id=33.

9. Jacob Yerushalmy and Herman Hilleboe, "Fat in the Diet and Mortality From Heart Disease; a Methodologic Note," *New York State Journal of Medicine* 57, no. 14 (1957): 2343-54.

10. Angus Maddison, "Economy Statistics: GDP Per Capita in 1950 (Most Recent) By Country," *NationMaster.com,* accessed June 12, 2013, http://www.nationmaster.com/graph/eco_gdp_per_cap_ in_195-economy-gdp-per-capita-1950. Israel and Ceylon/Sri Lanka omitted due to lack of recorded GDP.

11. Ancel Keys, *Seven Countries: A Multivariate Analysis of Death and Coronary Heart Disease* (Cambridge: Harvard University Press, 1980), v-vii.

12. "Health Revolutionary: The Life and Work of Ancel Keys," University of Minnesota School of Public Health, 2002, http://www. asph.org/movies/keys.pdf.

13. Keys, *Seven Countries,* 41.

14. Ibid., vi.

15. Ibid., 130.

16. Ibid.

17. Ibid.

18. Hisashi Adachi and Asuka Hino, "Trends in Nutritional Intake and Serum Cholesterol Levels Over 40 Years in Tanushimaru, Japan," *Journal of Epidemiology* 15, no. 3 (2005): 85-9.

19. Keys, *Seven Countries,* 123.

20. Constantine Vardavas et al., "Cardiovascular Disease Risk Factors and Dietary Habits of Farmers From Crete 45 Years After the First Description of the Mediterranean Diet," *European Journal of Preventive Cardiology* 17, no. 4 (2010): 440-6.

21. Keys, *Seven Countries*, 132.

22. Keys, *Seven Countries*, 131-132.

23. Sinikka Äijänseppä et al., "Serum Cholesterol and Depressive Symptoms in Elderly Finnish Men," *International Journal of Geriatric Psychiatry* 17, no. 7 (2002): 629-34.

24. Keys, *Seven Countries*, 124.

25. Ibid., 134.

26. Ibid., 124.

27. Ibid., 123.

28. Demosthenes Panagiotakos, et al., "Total Cholesterol and Body Mass Index in Relation to 40-Year Cancer Mortality (the Corfu Cohort of the Seven Countries Study)," *Cancer Epidemiology, Biomarkers, and Prevention* 14, no. 7 (2005): 1797-801.

29. Keys, *Seven Countries*, 135.

30. Ibid., 325.

31. Geoffrey Cannon, "Out of the Christmas Box," *Public Health Nutrition* 7, no. 8 (2004): 987-90.

32. "The Fasting Rule of the Orthodox Christian Church," Orthodox Saints and Feasts, accessed August 4, 2013, http://www.abbamoses.com/fasting.html.

33. "Fasting and Fast-Free Seasons of the Church," Orthodox Church in America, accessed August 3, 2013, http://oca.org/liturgics/outlines/fasting-fast-free-seasons-of-the-church.

34. Leonie K. Heilbronn et al., "Effect of 6-Month Calorie Restriction on Biomarkers of Longevity, Metabolic Adaptation, and Oxidative Stress in Overweight Individuals," *JAMA: The Journal of the American Medical Association* 295, no. 13 (2006): 1539-48.

35. Katerina Sarri et al., "Greek Orthodox Fasting Rituals: A Hidden Characteristic of the Mediterranean Diet of Crete," *British Journal of Nutrition* 92, no. 2 (2004): 277-284.

36. Katerina Sarri, Caroline Codrington, and Anthony Kafatos, "Does the Periodic Vegetarianism of Greek Orthodox Christians Benefit Blood Pressure?" *Preventative Medicine* 44, no. 4 (2007): 341-8.

37. Katerina Sarri et al., "Effects of Greek Orthodox Christian Church Fasting on Serum Lipids and Obesity," *BMC Public Health* 16, no. 3 (2003): 16.

38. Cannon, "Out of the Christmas Box."

39. Katerina Sarri and Anthony Kafatos, "The Seven Countries Study in Crete: Olive Oil, Mediterranean Diet or Fasting?" *Public Health Nutrition* 8, no. 6 (2005): 666.

40. Sohair al-Nagdy, D.S. Miller, R.U. Qureshi, and John Yudkin, "Metabolic Differences Between Starch and Sugar," *Nature* 209, no. 5018 (1966): 81-2.

41. John Yudkin and Janet Roddy, "Dietary Sucrose in Patients with Occlusive Atherosclerotic Disease," *Lancet* 284, no. 7349 (1964): 6-8.

42. John Yudkin, Pure, *White and Deadly* (London: Penguin Books, 1986), 91.

43. Ibid., 96 – 97.

44. Ibid., 97.

45. Ibid., 5.

46. Ibid., 8-9.

47. Rachel N. Carmody and Richard W. Wrangham, "The Energetic Significance of Cooking," *Journal of Human Evolution* 57, no. 4 (2009): 379-91.

48. Yudkin, *Pure, White and Deadly*, 3.

49. Ibid., 59.

50. Roberto Masironi, "Dietary Factors and Coronary Heart Disease," *Bulletin of the World Health Organization* 42, no. 1 (1970): 103-14.

51. Ibid.

52. Yudkin, *Pure, White and Deadly*, 86.

53. Ibid.

54. Ancel Keys, "Sucrose in the Diet and Coronary Heart Disease," *Atherosclerosis* 14, no. 2 (1971): 193-202.

55. Keys, *Seven Countries*, 253.

56. Christopher J. Burns-Cox, Richard Doll, and K. Ball, "Sugar Intake and Myocardial Infarction," *British Heart Journal* 31, no. 4 (1969): 485-90.

57. William B. Grant, "Commentary: Ecologic Studies in Identifying Dietary Risk Factors For Coronary Heart Disease and Cancer," *International Journal of Epidemiology* 37, no. 6 (2008): 1209-11.

58. Ancel Keys and Margaret Keys, *How to Eat Well and Stay Well: The Mediterranean Way* (Garden City, NY: Doubleday and Company, 1975), 58.

59. Ibid.
60. Ibid., 59.
61. Ibid.
62. Yudkin, *Pure, White and Deadly,* 79.
63. John Yudkin, "Diet and Coronary Heart Disease: Why Blame Fat?" *Journal of the Royal Society of Medicine* 85, no. 9 (1992): 515-6.
64. Yudkin, *Pure, White and Deadly,* 79-80.
65. Ibid., 5.
66. Ibid., 99.
67. Ibid., 100.
68. John Yudkin, "Carbohydrate Confusion," *Journal of the Royal Society of Medicine* 71, no. 8 (1978): 551-6.
69. Remko Kuipers et al.,"Saturated Fat, Carbohydrates and Cardiovascular Disease," *Netherlands Journal of Medicine* 69, no. 9 (2011): 372-8.
70. Rosa Maria Corbo and R. Sacchi, "Apolipoprotein E (APOE) Allele Distribution in the World. Is APOE*4 a "Thrifty" Allele?" *Annals of Human Genetics* 63, no. 4 (1999): 301-10.
71. Charlotte Hanlon and David Rubinsztein, "Arginine Residues at Condons 112 and 158 in the Apolipoprotein Gene Correspond to the Ancestral State in Humans," *Atherosclerosis* 112, no. 1 (1995): 85-90.
72. Annick McIntosh et al., "The Apolipoprotein E (APOE) Gene Appears Functionally Monomorphic in Chimpanzees *(Pan troglodytes),*" *PLoS ONE* 7, no. 10: e47760.
73. Joshua Fainman et al., "A Primate Model for Alzheimer's Disease: Investigation of the Apolipoprotein E Profile of the Vervet Monkey of St. Kitts," *American Journal of Medical Genetics Part B: Neuropsychiatric Genetics* 5, no. 144B (2007): 818-9.
74. Stephanie Fullerton et al., "Apolipoprotein E Variation at the Sequence Haplotype Level: Implications for the Origins and Maintenance of a Major Human Polymorphism," *American Journal of Human Genetics* 67, no. 4 (2000): 881-900.
75. Yiqing Song, Meir Stampfer, and Simin Liu, "Meta-Analysis: Apolipoprotein E Genotypes and Risk for Coronary Heart Disease," *Annals of Internal Medicine* 141, no. 2 (2004): 137-47.

76. Hannia Campos, Michael D'Agostino, and José M. Ordovás, "Gene-Diet Interactions and Plasma Lipoproteins: Role of Apoliporpotein E and Habitual Saturated Fat Intake," *Genetic Epidemiology* 20, no. 1 (2001): 117-28.

77. Laia Jofre-Monseny, Anne-Marie Minihane, and Gerald Rimbach, "Impact of ApoE Genotype on Oxidative Stress, Inflammation and Disease Risk," *Molecular Nutrition and Food Research* 52, no. 1 (2008): 131-145.

78. Yadong Yang et al., "Effect of Apolipoprotein E Genotype and Saturated Fat Intake on Plasma Lipids and Myocardial Infarction in the Central Valley of Costa Rica," *Human Biology* 79, no. 6 (2007): 637-47.

79. Ancel Keys, "Human Atherosclerosis and the Diet," *Circulation* 5, no. 1 (1952): 115-8.

80. Ancel Keys, Joseph Anderson, and Francisco Grande, "Serum Cholesterol Response to Changes in the Diet: II. The Effect of Cholesterol in the Diet," *Metabolism* 14, no. 7 (1965): 759-65.

81. Keys, *Seven Countries*, 194-195.

82. Ibid.

83. "Shades of Grey," *Nature* 497, no. 7450 (2013): 410.

84. Ibid.

85. "Interview With Walter Willet, M.D.," *Diet Wars,* Frontline PBS, January 9, 2004, http://www.pbs.org/wgbh/pages/frontline/shows/diet/interviews/willett.html.

86. "Healthy Eating Plate and Healthy Eating Pyramid," *The Nutrition Source,* Harvard School of Public Health, accessed August 30, 2013, http://www.hsph.harvard.edu/nutritionsource/pyramid/.

87. Ibid.

88. "Interview With Walter Willet, M.D," *Diet Wars.*

89. David M. Burns et al., "Cigarette Smoking Behavior in the United States," in *Monograph 8: Changes in Cigarette-Related Disease Risks and Their Implications for Prevention and Control,* Cancer Control and Population Sciences, National Cancer Institute, last updated May 21, 2013, http://cancercontrol.cancer.gov/brp/tcrb/monographs/8/m8_2.pdf.

90. Daniel Yam, Abraham Eliraz, and Elliot M. Berry, "Diet and Disease—the Israeli Paradox: Possible Dangers of a High Omega-6 Polyunsaturated Fatty Acid Diet," *Israel Journal of Medical Sciences* 32, no. 11 (1996): 1134-43.
91. Yudkin, *Pure, White and Deadly,* 168.
92. Ibid., 169.

8. A Little Town in Massachusetts

1. William P. Castelli, "Concerning the Possibility of a Nut," *JAMA Internal Medicine* 152, no. 7 (1992): 1371-2.
2. Michael Greger, "Accusation #15: AtkinsFacts.org Makes 'Misleading' Assertion About Saturated Fat," *AtkinsExposed.org,* accessed June 19, 2013, http://www.atkinsexposed.org/atkins/196/Atkins_Corporation_Mislabels_and_Misleads.htm.
3. Castelli, "Concerning the Possibility of a Nut."
4. William B. Kannel and Tavia Gordon, "Section 24: The Framingham diet study: Diet and the regulation of serum cholesterol," in *The Framingham Study: An Epidemiological Investigation of Cardiovascular Diseases* (Washington, D.C.: US Government Printing Office, 1970).
5. Hannia Campos et al., "LDL Particle Size Distribution: Results From the Framingham Offspring Study," *Arteriosclerosis and Thrombosis* 12, no. 12 (1992): 1410-9.
6. Barbara Millen Posner et al., "Diet, Menopause, and Serum Cholesterol Levels in Women: The Framingham Study," *American Heart Journal* 125, no. 2 (1993): 483-9.
7. Thomas R. Dawber, Rita J. Nickerson, Frederick N. Brand, and Jeremy Pool, "Eggs, Serum Cholesterol, and Coronary Heart Disease," *American Journal of Clinical Nutrition* 36, no. 4 (1982): 617-25.
8. Barbara Millen Posner et al., "Dietary Lipid Predictors of Coronary Heart Disease in Men. The Framingham Study," *Archives of Internal Medicine* 151, no. 6 (1991): 1181-7.
9. Matthew W. Gillman et al., "Inverse Association of Dietary Fat With Development of Ischemic Stroke in Men," *Journal of the American Medical Association* 278, no. 24 (1997): 2145-50.
10. Mary J. Emond and Wojciech Zareba, "Prognostic Value of Cholesterol in Women of Different Ages," *Journal of Women's Health* 6, no. 3 (1997): 295-307.

11. Ibid.

12. Paul D. Sorlie and Manning Feinleib, "The Serum Cholesterol-Cancer Relationship: An Analysis of Time Trends in the Framingham Study," *Journal of the National Cancer Institute* 69, no. 5 (1982): 989-96.

13. Bernard E. Kreger et al., "Serum Cholesterol Level, Body Mass Index, and the Risk of Colon Cancer: The Framingham Study," *Cancer* 70, no. 5 (1992): 1038-43.

14. Penelope K. Elias et al., "Serum Cholesterol and Cognitive Performance in the Framingham Heart Study," *Psychosomatic Medicine* 67, no. 1 (2005): 24-30.

9. PUFA-rama: The Rise of Vegetable Oils

1. "Our History—How it Began," *P&G,* accessed January 12, 2013, http://www.pg.com/en_US/downloads/media/Fact_Sheets_CompanyHistory.pdf.

2. Upton Sinclair, *The Jungle* (New York: Doubleday, Page and Company, 1906), 102.

3. Bryan Hayes, "Upton Sinclair's 'The Jungle' Turns 100," *PBS NewsHour,* May 10, 2006, http://www.pbs.org/newshour/extra/features/jan-june06/jungle_5-10.html.

4. "The Month," *The Westminster Review* 166, (July 1906): 365, http://www.archive.org/stream/westminsterrevi01wasogoog/westminsterrevi01wasogoog_djvu.txt.

5. Gary List and Michael Jackson, "Giants of the Past: The Battle Over Hydrogenation (1903-1920)," National Center for Agricultural Utilization Research, July 1, 2007, http://www.ars.usda.gov/research/publications/publications.htm?seq_no_115=210614.

6. Susan C. Pendleton, "'Man's Most Important Food is Fat:' The Use of Persuasive Techniques in Procter & Gamble's Public Relations Campaign to Introduce Crisco, 1911-1913," *Public Relations Quarterly* 44, no. 1 (1999): 6.

7. List and Jackson, "Giants of the Past."

8. "Historical Perspectives on Vegetable Oil-Based Diesel Fuels," *Inform* 12, no. 11 (2001): 1103-7.

9. Barbara Jennings, "Dr. Otto's Amazing Oil," Pennsylvania Center for the Book, Penn State University Library, Fall 2010, http://pabook.libraries.psu.edu/palitmap/Cottonseed.html.

10. Elsimar Metzker Coutinho, "Gossypol: A Contraceptive for Men," *Contraception* 65, no. 4 (2002): 259-63.

11. List and Jackson, "Giants of the Past."

12. Pendleton, "'Man's Most Important Food is Fat.'"

13. Marion Harris Neil, *The Story of Crisco* (Hong Kong: Forgotten Books, 2013), 10.

14. Neil, *The Story of Crisco,* 19.

15. Stephen Guyenet, "Butter, Margarine and Heart Disease," *Whole Health Source* (blog), December 27, 2008, http://wholehealthsource.blogspot.com/2008/12/butter-margarine-and-heart-disease.html.

16. David Schleifer, "We Spent a Million Bucks and Then We Had to Do Something: The Unexpected Implications of Industry Involvement in Trans Fat Research," *Bulletin of Science, Technology and Society* 31, no. 6 (2011): 460-471.

17. Fred A. Kummerow, "Nutritional Effects of Isomeric Fats: Their Possible Influence on Cell Metabolism or Cell Structure," in *Dietary Fats and Health,* eds. Edward George Perkins and W.J Visek (Champaign, IL: American Oil Chemists' Society, 1983), 391-402.

18. *Dietary Goals for the United States—Supplemental Views* (Washington, D.C.: Government Printing Office, 1977), 139-40.

19. Luise Light, "The Education of an American—Part One," Rense. com, November 1, 2007, http://rense.com/general78/educa.htm.

20. Herbert Heckers and Franz W. Melcher, "Trans-Isomeric Fatty Acids Present in West German Margarines, Shortenings, Frying and Cooking Fats," *American Journal of Clinical Nutrition* 31, no. 6 (1978): 1041-9.

21. Light, "The Education of an American—Part One."

22. Alice H. Lichtenstein et al., "Diet and Lifestyle Recommendations Revision 2006: A Scientific Statement From the American Heart Association Nutrition Committee," *Circulation* 114, no. 1 (2006): 82-96.

23. Ronald P. Mensink and Martijn B. Katan, "Effect of Dietary Trans Fatty Acids on High-Density and Low-Density Lipoprotein Cholesterol Levels in Healthy Subjects," *New England Journal of Medicine* 323, no. 7 (1990): 439-45.

24. "The Food Guide Pyramid," *United States Department of Agriculture.*

25. Osmo Turpeinen et al., "Dietary Prevention of Coronary Heart Disease: The Finnish Mental Hospital Study," *International Journal of Epidemiology* 8, no. 2 (1979): 99-118.

26. Carl Lavie et al., "Omega-3 Polyunsaturated Fatty Acids and Cardiovascular Diseases," *Journal of the American College of Cardiology* 54, no. 7 (2009): 585-94.

27. Peter L. Zock, Jeanne H.M. de Vries, and Martijn B. Katan, "Impact of Myristic Acid Versus Palmitic Acid on Serum Lipid and Lipoprotein Levels in Healthy Women and Men," *Arteriosclerosis, Thrombosis, and Vascular Biology* 14, no. 4 (1994): 567-75.

28. Charlotte Cox et al., "Effects of Coconut Oil, Butter, and Safflower Oil on Lipids and Lipoproteins in Persons with Moderately Elevated Cholesterol Levels," *Journal of Lipid Research* 36, no. 8 (1995): 1787-95.

29. Christopher E. Ramsden, Joseph R. Hibbeln, Sharon F. Majchrzak, and John M. Davis, "N-6 Fatty Acid-Specific and Mixed Polyunsaturate Dietary Interventions Have Different Effects on CHD Risk: A Meta-Analysis of Randomised Controlled Trials," *British Journal of Nutrition* 104, no. 11 (2010): 1586-1600.

30. Matti Miettinen et al., "Cholesterol-Lowering Diet and Mortality From Coronary Heart Disease," *Lancet* 300, no. 7792 (1972): 1418-9.

31. Wayne A. Ray and Keith G. Meador, "Antipsychotics and Sudden Death: is Thioridazine the Only Bad Actor?" *British Journal of Psychiatry* 180, (2002): 483-4.

32. Paul Leren, "The Effect of Plasma Cholesterol Lowering Diet in Male Survivors of Myocardial Infarction. A Controlled Clinical Trial," *Acta Medica Scandinavica Supplementum* 446, (1966): 1-92.

33. Ibid.

34. Ibid., 27-8.

35. Ramsden et al., "N-6 Fatty Acid-Specific and Mixed Polyunsaturate Dietary Interventions Have Different Effects on CHD Risk: A Meta-Analysis of Randomised Controlled Trials."

36. Ibid.

37. Morton Lee Pearce and Seymour Dayton, "Incidence of Cancer in Men on a Diet High in Polyunsaturated Fat," *Lancet* 297, no. 7697 (1971): 464-7.

38. S. Duncan, "Pledge Award Winner: SDA Soybean Development Provides a Sustainable Source of Omega-3," Monsanto, July 13, 2009, http://www.monsanto.com/newsviews/Pages/Pledge-Award-SDA-Soybean-Sustainable-Source-Omega-3.aspx.

39. William S. Harris et al., "Stearidonic Acid-Enriched Soybean Oil Increased the Omega-3 Index, an Emerging Cardiovascular Risk Marker," *Lipids* 43, no. 9 (2008): 805-11.

40. Shawna L. Lemke et al., "Dietary Intake of Stearidonic Acid-Enriched Soybean Oil Increases the Omega-3 Index: Randomized, Double-Blind Clinical Study of Efficacy and Safety," *American Journal of Clinical Nutrition* 92, no. 4 (2010): 766-75.

41. William S. Harris, "Stearidonic Acid as a 'Pro-Eicosapentaenoic Acid,'" *Current Opinion in Lipidology* 23, no. 1 (2012): 30-4.

42. Philip C. Calder, "The American Heart Association Advisory on N-6 Fatty Acids: Evidence Based or Biased Evidence?" *British Journal of Nutrition* 104, no. 11 (2010): 1575-6.

43. "Report of the Cardiovascular Review Group of the Committee on Medical Aspects of Food Policy (COMA)," in *Nutritional Aspects of Cardiovascular Disease, Report on Health and Social Subjects,* no. 46 (London: The Stationery Office, 1994).

44. Shelley Wood, "AHA Champions Omega-6 PUFAs to Counter Popular Nutrition Advice," TheHeart.org, accessed January 13, 2012, http://www.theheart.org/article/937865.do.

45. Francesco Sofi et al., "Dietary Habits, Lifestyle and Cardiovascular Risk Factors in a Clinically Healthy Italian Population: the "Florence" Diet is Not Mediterranean," *European Journal of Clinical Nutrition* 59, no. 4 (2005): 584-91.

46. Ibid.

47. "KFC Sued for Fouling Chicken with Partially Hydrogenated Oil," Center for Science in the Public Interest, June 12, 2006, http://www.cspinet.org/new/200606121.html.

10. Meet Your Meat

1. Kerin O'Dea, "Traditional Diet and Food Preferences of Australian Aboriginal Hunter-Gatherers," *Philosophical Transactions of the Royal Society of London; Series B: Biological Sciences* 334, no. 1270 (1991): 240-1.

2. Helga Refsum and Per Ueland, "Homocysteine and Cardiovascular Disease," *Annual Review of Medicine* 49, (1998): 31-62.

3. Reinald Pamplona and Gustavo Barja, "Mitochondrial Oxidative Stress, Aging, and Caloric Restriction: the Protein and Methionine Connection," *Biochimica et Biophysica Acta* 1757, no. 5-6 (2006): 496-508.

4. Takashi Sugimura et al., "Heterocyclic Amines: Mutagens/Carcinogens Produced During Cooking of Meat and Fish," *Cancer Science* 95, no. 4 (2004): 290-9.

5. Nobuyuki Ito et al., "A New Colon and Mammary Carcinogen in Cooked Food, 2-Amino-1-Methyl-6-Phenylimidazo[4,5-b] Pyridine (PhlP)," *Carcinogenesis* 12, no. 8 (1991): 1503-6.

6. Tamami Kato et al., "Carcinogenicity in Rats of a Mutagenic Compound, 2-Amino-3,8-Dimethylimidazo[4,5-f]Quinoxaline," *Carcinogenesis* 9, no. 1 (1988): 71-3.

7. Tamami Kato et al., "Induction of Tumors in the Zymbal Gland, Oral Cavity, Colon, Skin and Mammary Gland of F344 Rats by a Mutagenic Compound, 2-Amino-3,4-Dimethylimidazo[4,5-f] Quinoline," *Carcinogenesis* 10, no. 3 (1989): 601-3.

8. Hiroko Ohgaki et al., "Carcinogenicity in Mice of a Mutagenic Compound, 2-Amino-3-Methylimidazo[4,5-f]Quinoline, from Broiled Sardine, Cooked Beef and Beef Extract," *Carcinogenesis* 5, no. 7 (1984): 921-4.

9. *Diet, Nutrition, and Cancer* (Washington, D.C.: National Academy Press, 1982), 1.

10. Marie Cantwell et al., "Relative Validity of a Food Frequency Questionnaire with a Meat-Cooking and Heterocyclic Amine Module," *Cancer Epidemiology, Biomarkers and Prevention* 13, no. 2 (2004): 293-8.

11. Shigeo Manabe, "Carcinogenic Heterocyclic Amines in the Environment," *Nihon Eiseigaku Zasshi* 46, no. 4 (1991): 867-73.

12. Kristin E. Anderson et al., "Meat Intake and Cooking Techniques: Associations with Pancreatic Cancer," *Mutation Research* 30, no. 506-7 (2002): 225-31.

13. Rashmi Sinha et al., "Meat, Meat Cooking Methods and Preservation, and Risk for Colorectal Adenoma," *Cancer Research* 65, no. 17 (2005): 8034-41.

14. Amanda J. Cross et al., "A Prospective Study of Meat and Meat Mutagens and Prostate Cancer Risk," *Cancer Research* 65, no. 24 (2005): 11779-84.

15. Armindo Melo et al., "Effect of Beer/Red Wine Marinades on the Formation of Heterocyclic Aromatic Amines in Pan-Fried Beef," *Journal of Agricultural and Food Chemistry* 56, no. 22 (2008): 10625-32.

16. Monika Gibis, "Effect of Oil Marinades With Garlic, Onion, and Lemon Juice on the Formation of Heterocyclic Aromatic Amines in Fried Beef Patties," *Journal of Agricultural and Food Chemistry* 55, no. 25 (2007): 10240-7.

17. Cynthia P. Salmon, Mark G. Knize, and James S. Felton, "Effects of Marinating on Heterocyclic Amine Carcinogen Formation in Grilled Chicken," *Food and Chemical Toxicology* 35, no. 5 (1997): 433-41.

18. Brian K. Crownover and Carlton J. Covey, "Hereditary Hemochromatosis," *American Family Physician* 87, no. 3 (2013): 183-90.

19. Leif Hallberg and Lena Rossander, "Effect of Different Drinks on the Absorption of Non-Heme Iron From Composite Meals," *Human Nutrition; Applied Nutrition* 36, no. 2 (1982): 116-23.

20. Yuichi Nakazawa et al., "On Stone-Boiling Technology in the Upper Paleolithic: Behavioral Implications From an Early Magdalenian Hearth in El Mirón Cave, Cantabria, Spain," *Journal of Archaeological Science* 36, no. 3 (2009): 684-693.

11. Herbivore's Dilemma

1. "Clinton's Weight Loss Secret: Plants," *The Situation Room*, CNN, September 21, 2010, http://edition.cnn.com/video/#/video/us/2010/09/21/intv.clinton.blitzer.weight.loss.cnn?hpt=C2.

2. (RH November 25, 1884; cited in 1Bio 30-31)

3. Gregory Holmes and Delbert Hodder, "Ellen G. White and the Seventh Day Adventist Church: Visions or Partial Complex Seizures?" *Journal of Neurology* 31, no. 4: 160-1.

4. Roger W. Coon, "Ellen G. White and Vegetarianism," *Ministry Magazine* 59, no. 4 (1986): 4-7.
5. Ellen G. White, *Testimony Studies on Diet and Food* (Ellen G. White Estate, 2010), http://www.anym.org/SOP/en_TSDF.pdf.
6. Ellen G. White, *Counsels on Diet and Foods* (Hagerstown, MD: Review and Herald Publishing, 1946), 291.
7. Elizabeth Free and Theodore M. Brown, "John Harvey Kellogg, MD: Health Reformer and Antismoking Crusader," *American Journal of Public Health* 92, no. 6 (2002): 935.
8. "The Adventist Health Study: Mortality Studies of Seventh-Day Adventists," Loma Linda University School of Public Health, accessed July 14, 2013, http://www.llu.edu/public-health/health/mortality.page.
9. Gary E. Fraser, "Associations Between Diet and Cancer, Ischemic Heart Disease, and All-Cause Mortality in Non-Hispanic White California Seventh-Day Adventists," *American Journal of Clinical Nutrition* 70, no. 3 (1999): 532s-8s.
10. James E. Enstrom, "Cancer Mortality Among Mormons," *Cancer* 36, no. 3 (1975):825-41.
11. Joseph L. Lyon, Harry P. Wetzler, John W. Gardner, Melville R. Klauber, and Roger R. Williams, "Cardiovascular Mortality in Mormons and Non-Mormons in Utah, 1969-1971," *American Journal of Epidemiology* 108, no. 5 (1978): 357-66.
12. Joseph L. Lyon et al., "Cancer Incidence in Mormons and Non-Mormons in Utah, 1966-1970," *New England Journal of Medicine* 294, no. 3 (1976): 129-33.
13. Joseph L. Lyon, John W. Gardner, and Dee W. West, "Cancer Incidence in Mormons and Non-Mormons in Utah During 1967-75," *Journal of the National Cancer Institute* 65, no. 5 (1980): 1055-61.
14. Gary E. Fraser and David J. Shavlik, "Ten Years of Life: Is It a Matter of Choice?" *JAMA Internal Medicine* 161, no. 13 (2001): 1645-52.
15. James E. Enstrom, "Cancer and Total Mortality Among Active Mormons," *Cancer* 42, no. 4 (1978): 1943-51.
16. Maria Gacek, "Selected Lifestyle and Health Condition Indices of Adults With Varied Models of Eating," *Roczniki Panstwowego Zakladu Higieny* 61, no. 1 (2010): 65-9.

17. Fraser, "Associations Between Diet and Cancer, Ischemic Heart Disease, and All-Cause Mortality in Non-Hispanic White California Seventh-Day Adventists."

18. Gacek, "Selected Lifestyle and Health Condition Indices of Adults With Varied Models of Eating."

19. Ibid.

20. Joan Sabaté, "The Contribution of Vegetarian Diets to Human Health," *Forum of Nutrition* 56, (2003): 218-20.

21. Claire T. McEvoy, Norman Temple, and Jayne V. Woodside, "Vegetarian Diets, Low-Meat Diets and Health: a Review," *Public Health Nutrition* 15, no. 12 (2012): 2287-94.

22. Dan Buettner, *The Blue Zones: Lessons for Living Longer From the People Who've Lived the Longest* (Washington, D.C. National Geographic, 2009).

23. Jenny Chang-Claude et al., "Lifestyle Determinants and Mortality in German Vegetarians and Health-Conscious Persons: Results of a 21-Year Follow-up," *Cancer Epidemiology, Biomarkers, and Prevention* 14, no. 4 (2005): 963-8.

24. Timothy J. Key et al., "Mortality in British vegetarians: review and preliminary results from EPIC-Oxford," *American Journal of Clinical Nutrition* 78, no. 3 (2003): 533S-8S.

25. Timothy J. Key, Margaret Thorogood, Paul N. Appleby, and Michael L. Burr, "Dietary Habits and Mortality in 11,000 Vegetarians and Health Conscious People: Results of a 17 Year Follow Up," *British Medical Journal* 313, no. 7060 (1996): 775-9.

26. Mats Lambe et al., "Parity, Age at First and Last Birth, and Risk of Breast Cancer: A Population-Based Study in Sweden," *Breast Cancer Research and Treatment* 38, no. 3 (1996): 305-11.

27. Key et al., "Mortality in British vegetarians: review and preliminary results from EPIC-Oxford."

28. David S. Martin, "From Omnivore to Vegan: The Dietary Education of Bill Clinton," *CNN Health,* August 18, 2011, http://www.cnn.com/2011/HEALTH/08/18/bill.clinton.diet.vegan/.

29. Dean Ornish et al., "Intensive Lifestyle Changes for Reversal of Coronary Heart Disease," *Journal of the American Medical Association* 280, no 23. (1998): 2001-7.

30. Caldwell B. Esselstyn, Jr. et al., "A Strategy to Arrest and Reverse Coronary Artery Disease: A 5-Year Longitudinal Study of a Single Physician's Practice," *Journal of Family Practice* 41, no. 6 (1995): 560-8.

31. Caldwell B. Esselstyn, Jr., "Updating A 12-Year Experience With Arrest and Reversal Therapy for Coronary Heart Disease (an Overdue Requiem for Palliative Cardiology)," *American Journal of Cardiology* 84, no. 3 (1999): 339-41, A8.

32. Neal D. Barnard et al., "A Low-Fat Vegan Diet and a Conventional Diabetes Diet in the Treatment of Type 2 Diabetes: a Randomized, Controlled, 74-Week Clinical Trial," *American Journal of Clinical Nutrition* 89, no. 5 (2009): 1588S-96S.

33. Ann Gibbons, "Bonobos Join Chimps and Closest Human Relatives," *Science,* June 13, 2012, http://news.sciencemag.org/sciencenow/2012/06/bonobo-genome-sequenced.html.

34. Milton R. Mills, "The Comparative Anatomy of Eating," *Vegsource.com,* November 21, 2009, http://www.vegsource.com/news/2009/11/the-comparative-anatomy-of-eating.html.

35. Kathy Freston, "Shattering the Meat Myth: Humans are Natural Vegetarians," *HuffPost Healthy Living,* June 11, 2009, http://www.huffingtonpost.com/kathy-freston/shattering-the-meat-myth_b_214390.html.

36. "The Natural Human Diet," *PETA.org,* accessed June 13, 2013, http://www.peta.org/living/vegetarian-living/the-natural-human-diet.aspx

37. Katharine Milton, "Nutritional Characteristics of Wild Primate Foods: Do the Diets of Our Closet Living Relatives Have Lessons for Us?" *Nutrition* 15, no. 6 (1999): 488-98.

38. Peter J. Van Soest, *Nutritional Ecology of the Ruminant* (Ithaca: Cornell University Press, 1982), 72.

39. David G. Popovich et al., "The Western Lowland Gorilla Diet Has Implications for the Health of Humans and Other Hominoids," *Journal of Nutrition* 127, no. 10 (1997): 2000-5.

40. Lara Pizzorno, "Common Genetic Variants and other Host-Related Factors Greatly Increase Susceptibility to Vitamin A Deficiency," *Longevity Medicine Review,* March 7, 2010, http://www.lmreview.com/articles/view/common-genetic-variants-and-other-host-related-factors-greatly-increase-susceptibility-to-vitamin-a-deficiency.

41. Pieter C. Dagnelie, Wija A. van Staveren, and Henk van den Berg, "Vitamin B-12 From Algae Appears Not to Be Bioavailable," *American Journal of Clinical Nutrition* 53, no. 3 (1991): 695-7.

42. Jerry L. Rosenblum and C.L Irwin, and David Hershel Alpers, "Starch and Glucose Oligosaccharides Protect Salivary-Type Amylase Activity at Acid pH," *American Journal of Physiology* 254, no. 5.1 (1988): G775-80.

43. John McDougall and Mary McDougall, *The Starch Solution: Eat the Foods You Love, Regain Your Health, and Lose the Weight for Good* (New York: Rodale Books, 2012), 13.

44. Abigail L. Mandel and Paul A.S. Breslin, "High Endogenous Salivary Amylase Activity is Associated with Improved Glycemic Homeostasis Following Starch Ingestion in Adults," *Journal of Nutrition* 142, no. 5 (2012): 853-8.

45. George H. Perry et al., "Diet and the Evolution of Human Amylase Gene Copy Number Variation," *Nature Genetics* 39, no. 10 (2007): 1256-60.

46. Ibid.

47. Verena Behringer et al., "Measurements of Salivary Alpha Amylase and Salivary Cortisol in Hominoid Primates Reveal Within-Species Consistency and Between-Species Differences," *PLoS ONE* 8, no. 4 (2013): e60773.

48. Marcus Mau et al., "Indication of Higher Salivary Alpha-Amylase Expression in Hamadryas Baboons and Geladas Compared to Chimpanzees and Humans," *Journal of Primatology* 39, no. 3 (2010): 187-90.

49. Perry et al., "Diet and the Evolution of Human Amylase Gene Copy Number Variation."

50. Mandel and Breslin, "High Endogenous Salivary Amylase Activity is Associated with Improved Glycemic Homeostasis Following Starch Ingestion in Adults."

12. A Future Informed by the Past

1. Staffan Lindeberg et al., "A Palaeolithic Diet Improves Glucose Tolerance More than a Mediterranean-Like Diet in Individuals With Ischaemic Heart Disease," *Diabetologia* 50, no. 9 (2007): 1795-807.

2. Tommy Jönsson et al., "Beneficial Effects of a Paleolithic Diet on Cardiovascular Risk Factors in Type 2 Diabetes: a Randomized Cross-Over Pilot Study," *Cardiovascular Diabetology* 8, no. 35 (2009).

3. Kerin O'Dea, "Marked Improvement in Carbohydrate and Lipid Metabolism in Diabetic Australian Aborigines after Temporary Reversion to Traditional Lifestyle," *Diabetes* 33, no. 6 (1984): 596-603.

4. Tommy Jönsson et al., "Subjective Satiety and Other Experiences of a Paleolithic Diet Compared to a Diabetes Diet in Patients With Type 2 Diabetes," *Nutrition Journal* 12, (2013): 105.

5. M. Osterdahl et al., "Effects of a Short-Term Intervention With a Paleolithic Diet in Healthy Volunteers," *European Journal of Clinical Nutrition* 62, no. 5 (2008): 682-5.

6. O'Dea, "Marked Improvement in Carbohydrate and Lipid Metabolism in Diabetic Australian Aborigines after Temporary Reversion to Traditional Lifestyle."

7. Heidi Ledford, "A Genetic Gift for Sushi Eaters: Seaweed-Rich Diet Leaves Its Mark on Gut Microbes," *Nature News,* April 7, 2010, http://www.nature.com/news/2010/100407/full/news.2010.169.html.

8. Esselstyn, Jr. et al, "A Strategy to Arrest and Reverse Coronary Artery Disease: A 5-Year Longitudinal Study of a Single Physician's Practice."

9. Dean Ornish et al., "Can Lifestyle Changes Reverse Coronary Heart Disease? The Lifestyle Heart Trial," *Lancet* 336, no. 8708 (1990): 129-33.

10. Barnard et al., "A Low-Fat Vegan Diet and a Conventional Diabetes Diet in the Treatment of Type 2 Diabetes: a Randomized, Controlled, 74-Week Clinical Trial."

11. Jens Kjeldsen-Kragh et al., "Controlled Trial of Fasting and One-Year Vegetarian Diet in Rheumatoid Arthritis," *Lancet* 338, no. 8772 (1991): 899-902.

12. Ann-Charlotte Elkan et al., "Gluten-Free Vegan Diet Induces Decreased LDL and Oxidized LDL Levels and Raised Athero-protective Natural Antibodies Against Phosphorylcholine in Patients With Rheumatoid Arthritis: a Randomized Study," *Arthritis Research and Therapy* 10, no. 2 (2008): R34.

13. Lluís Serra-Majem, Blanca Roman, and Ramón Estruch, "Scientific Evidence of Interventions Using the Mediterranean Diet," *Nutrition Reviews* 64, no. 2.2 (2006): S27-47.

14. "The Island Where People Live Longer," NPR, May 2, 2009, http://www.npr.org/templates/story/story.php?storyId=103744881.

15. Antonia Trichopoulou et al., "Nutritional Composition and Flavonoid Content of Edible Greens and Green Pies: a Potential Rich Source of Antioxidant Nutrients in the Mediterranean Diet," *Food Chemistry* 70, no. 3 (2000): 319-323.

16. Sabrina Zeghichi, Stamatina Kallithraka, Artemis P. Simopoulos, and Zaxarias Kypriotakis, "Nutritional Composition of Selected Wild Plants in the Diet," *World Review of Nutrition and Dietetics* 91, (2003): 22-40.

17. Constantine I. Vardavas et al., "The Antioxidant and Phylloquinone Content of Wildly Grown Greens in Crete," *Food Chemistry* 99, no. 4 (2006): 813-821.

18. Antonia Trichopoulou, Androniki Naska, and Effie Vasilopoulou, "Guidelines for the Intake of Vegetables and Fruit: the Mediterranean Approach," *International Journal for Vitamin and Nutrition Research* 71, no. 3 (2001): 149-53.

19. Lindeberg et al., "A Palaeolithic Diet Improves Glucose Tolerance More than a Mediterranean-Like Diet in Individuals With Ischaemic Heart Disease."

20. Weston A. Price, *Nutrition and Physical Degeneration*, 6th edition (La Mesa, CA: Price-Pottenger Nutrition Foundation, 2003), 472.

21. Ibid., chapter 18.

22. Ibid., introduction.

23. Ibid., chapter 6.

24. Ibid.

25. Ibid., chapter 9.

26. Ibid., chapter 11.

27. Ibid., chapter 9.

28. Ibid., chapter 3.

29. Ibid., chapter 15.

30. Ibid., chapter 4.

31. Ibid., chapter 15.

32. Ibid., chapter 5.

33. Ibid., chapter 15.

34. Ibid., chapter 6.

35. Ibid., chapter 15.

36. Ibid., chapter 7.

37. Ibid., chapter 8.

38. Ibid., chapter 15.

39. Ibid., chapter 9.

40. Ibid., chapter 15.

41. Ibid., chapter 10.

42. Ibid., chapter 15.

43. Ibid., chapter 12.

44. Ibid., chapter 15.

45. Ibid.

46. Ibid., chapter 13.

47. Ibid., chapter 15.

48. Ibid.

49. Ibid.

50. Lindsey F. Masson, Geraldine McNeill, and Alison Avenell, "Genetic Variation and the Lipid Response to Dietary Intervention: a Systematic Review," *American Journal of Clinical Nutrition* 77, no. 5 (2003): 1098-111.

51. "Cutting Carbs is More Effective than Low-Fat Diet for Insulin-Resistant Women, Study Finds," *Science Daily,* June 21, 2010, http://www.sciencedaily.com/releases/2010/06/100619173919.htm.

52. Price, *Nutrition and Physical Degeneration,* chapter 21. Hat tip to Chris Masterjohn.

53. Karl E. Anderson et al., "Diet-Hormone Interactions: Protein/Carbohydrate Ratio Alters Reciprocally the Plasma Levels of Testosterone and Cortisol and Their Respective Binding Globulins in Man," *Life Sciences* 40, no. 18 (1987): 1761-8.

54. Elliot Danforth, Jr. et al, "Dietary-Induced Alterations in Thyroid Hormone Metabolism During Overnutrition," *Journal of Clinical Investigation* 64, no. 5 (1979): 1336-47.

List of Tables

List of Figures

Index

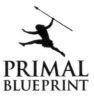

PRIMAL
BLUEPRINT

Other books by Primal Blueprint Publishing

MARK SISSON

 The Primal Connection: *Follow your genetic blueprint to health and happiness*

 The Primal Blueprint: *Reprogram your genes for effortless weight loss, vibrant health, and boundless energy*

 The Primal Blueprint 21-Day Total Body Transformation: *A step-by-step gene reprogramming action plan*

 The Primal Blueprint 90-Day Journal: *A Personal Experiment (n=1)*

COOKBOOKS BY MARK SISSON AND JENNIFER MEIER

 The Primal Blueprint Cookbook: *Primal, low carb, paleo, grain-free, dairy-free and gluten-free meals*

 The Primal Blueprint Quick and Easy Meals: *Delicous, Primal-approved meals you can make in under 30 minutes*

 The Primal Blueprint Healthy Sauces, Dressings, and Toppings: *Plus rubs, dips, marinades and other easy ways to transform basic natural foods into Primal masterpieces*

PRIMAL
BLUEPRINT

Other books by Primal Blueprint Publishing

OTHER AUTHORS

Hidden Plague: *A field guide for surviving and overcoming Hidradenitis Suppurativa,* by Tara Grant

Rich Food, Poor Food: *The Ultimate Grocery Purchasing System (GPS),* by Mira Calton, CN, and Jayson Calton, Ph.D.

COOKBOOKS

The Paleo Primer: *A jump-start guide to losing body fat and living Primally,* by Keris Marsden and Matt Whitmore

Primal Cravings: *Your favorite foods made Paleo,* by Brandon and Megan Keatley